Health Technical Memorandum 2007

Design considerations

Electrical services supply and distribution

London : HMSO

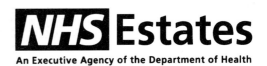

An Executive Agency of the Department of Health

ISBN 0 11 321685 8

HMSO
Standing order service

Placing a standing order with HMSO BOOKS enables a
customer to receive future titles in this series automatically
as published. This saves the time, trouble and expense of
placing individual orders and avoids the problem of
knowing when to do so. For details please write to HMSO
BOOKS (PC 13A/1), Publications Centre, PO Box 276,
London SW8 5DT quoting reference 14.02.017.
The standing order service also enables customers to receive
automatically as published all material of their choice which
additionally saves extensive catalogue research. The scope
and selectivity of the service has been extended by new
techniques, and there are more than 3,500 classifications to
choose from. A special leaflet describing the service in detail
may be obtained on request.

About this publication

Health Technical Memoranda (HTMs) give comprehensive advice and guidance on the design, installation and operation of specialised building and engineering technology used in the delivery of healthcare.

They are applicable to new and existing sites, and are of use at various stages during the inception, design, construction, refurbishment and maintenance of a building.

Health Technical Memorandum 2007

HTM 2007 focuses on the

a.   legal and mandatory requirements;

b.   design applications;

c.   maintenance;

d.   operation

of electrical services supply and distribution in all types of healthcare and personal social services premises.

It is published as four separate volumes, each addressing a specialist discipline:

- **Management policy** – outlines the overall responsibility of managers of healthcare and personal social services premises, and details their legal and mandatory obligations in setting up and operating reliable, efficient and economic electrical services. It summarises the technical aspects involved and concludes with a list of definitions;

- this volume – **Design considerations** – details the requirements and considerations that should be applied to the design of electrical services up to the contract document. Guidance is given on the choice of supply, distribution voltages, equipment, cabling and utilisation circuits. Typical system layout and sub-station/ switchroom configurations are also shown;

- **Validation and verification** – details the requirements for ensuring that manufactured equipment is formally tested and certified as to contract, and manufactured to the highest level of quality assurance. The importance of commissioning is emphasised and the order of tests on site is listed. Routine testing, which is a subset of these commissioning tests, is also reviewed;

- **Operational management** – provides information for those responsible for overseeing and operating day-to-day running and maintenance. Coverage includes routine tests, planned preventive maintenance and troubleshooting.

Guidance in this Health Technical Memorandum is complemented by the library of National Health Service Model Engineering Specifications. Users of the guidance are advised to refer to the relevant specifications for "Electrical services".

The contents of this Health Technical Memorandum in terms of management policy, operational policy and technical guidance are endorsed by:

a.	The Welsh Office for the NHS in Wales;

b.	The Health and Personal Social Services Management Executive in Northern Ireland;

c.	The National Health Service in Scotland Management Executive,

and they set standards consistent with Departmental Cost Allowances.

Statutory guidance on electrical safety to meet the Electricity at Work Regulations 1989 is published in HTM 2020 – 'Electrical safety code for low voltage systems' and HTM 2021 – 'Electrical safety code for high voltage systems'.

Guidance on emergency electrical requirements is published in HTM 2011 – 'Emergency electrical services'. Guidance on reduction of electrical interference is given in HTM 2014 – 'Abatement of electrical interference'.

References to legislation appearing in the main text of this guidance apply in England and Wales. Where references differ for Scotland and/or Northern Ireland, these are given as marginal notes.

Where appropriate, marginal notes are also used to amplify the text.

Contents

1.0 Scope

1.1 Electrical services form an integral part of the healthcare and personal social services premises (HCP) supply and distribution network in meeting both safety and functional requirements.

Nursing Homes & Agencies Act (Northern Ireland) 1971; Nursing Homes Regulations (Northern Ireland) 1974; Registered Establishments (Scotland) Act 1987

Electricity at Work Regulations (Northern Ireland), SI 191/13

1.2 The provision of electrical services in HCP is a management responsibility at both new and existing sites. This guidance is equally applicable to premises which offer acute healthcare services under the Registered Homes Act 1984.

1.3 This guidance also provides an insight into the requirements of the Electricity at Work Regulations 1989.

1.4 Healthcare and personal social services premises are totally dependent upon electrical power supplies, not only to maintain a safer and more comfortable environment for patients and staff, but also to give greater scope for treatment using sophisticated medical equipment at all levels of clinical and surgical care. Changes in application, design and statutory requirements have led to the introduction of a new generation of equipment and new standards of reliability; hence, a large expansion of material is included in the current HTM.

1.5 Interruptions in electrical power supplies to equipment can seriously disrupt the delivery of healthcare, with serious consequences for patient well-being. Healthcare and personal social services premises must therefore ensure that their electrical installation provides maximum reliability and integrity of supplies. Every effort must be made to reduce the probability of equipment failure due to loss of power from the regional electricity company and from internal emergency power sources.

2.0 Design of installations for growth and change

2.1 Subsequent additions to an installation, unless planned and allowed for during the original construction, can be costly, particularly when structural changes are involved. The aim should be to make adequate provision for known requirements, including spare capacity in transformers, cables, and bus-bars and, where practicable, to include suitable provision to enable the installation to be extended. It is important to note that an increase in cable size initially is relatively inexpensive compared to the cost of installing an additional cable later. The installation should be designed to be as flexible as possible within the cost limits, to allow for possible future additions and alterations.

3.0 Electrical supplies, tariffs and load factor

Tariffs

3.1   The type and choice of tariff available to HCP can vary considerably. Tariffs should be discussed at an early stage with the commercial engineer of a regional electricity company (REC) or any other supplier. The discussions should focus on preferential tariffs. Guarantees for the reliability and integrity of electrical supplies should be emphasised.

3.2   Normally, two basic types of tariffs are available. These are "block" or "maximum demand". There is a maximum limit for block tariffs and a minimum limit for maximum demand tariffs. These values vary with different electricity suppliers. Possible variations in both the basic types of tariff include reduced rates for off-peak (night and/or weekend) consumption.

Load factor

3.3   As far as practicable, the installation should be designed to cope with the variable load, spread over 24 hours, to obtain the optimum load factor and to take full advantage of any night and weekend rebates which are applicable.

4.0 Estimated maximum demand

4.1 The estimated maximum power demand will partly determine the capacity of the supply load rating and the location of main distribution equipment.

4.2 The maximum power demand in kW and maximum load in kVA, together with the method of distribution, will influence negotiations on the final tariff agreed.

4.3 Among the factors which will increase maximum demands are deep plan designed buildings which require higher standards of illumination and mechanical ventilation.

4.4 To obtain the installation maximum demand, load schedules are required, together with details of equipment. If details of subsequent construction phases are not available, it is necessary to estimate the ultimate maximum demand using available information relating to the complete project.

4.5 A survey of electricity bills from 1507 HCPs carried out in 1988/89 provides an insight into typical maximum demands. In all these HCPs space heating was mainly non-electric. Table 1 shows a summary of maximum demands pertaining to various HCP classifications:

  a. column 1 – HCPs classified by type no;

  b. column 2 – HCP description;

  c. column 3 – building volume heated by non-electric means;

  d. column 4 – number of electricity bills per class of HCP;

  e. column 5 – load range;

  f. column 6 – statistical derivation of maximum demand.

1 HCP classification by type number	2 Description	3 Size $\times$ 100 m^3	4 No of bills	5 Load range*	6 Stat*
01,02,03,17	Acute	<150	143	168–14, 142	1242
01,02,03,17	Acute	150–600	108	43–7819	1243
01,02,03,17	Acute	>600	186	131–10, 103	1133
04, 05	Long stay	—	117	98–6315	967
11	Maternity	—	20	231–987	976
12,13	Mental illness	<300	121	188–11,367	1178
12,13	Mental illness	>300	103	131–6003	722
14	Orthopaedic	—	14	267–3372	1206
19	Other hospitals	—	49	165–2875	1166

Total number of HCPs sampled, 1507. Designers of HCP electrical services can use the figures in column 6 to satisfy 90% of the individual HCP classification

Table 1 DH (NHS Estates) energy data system – maximum demand by HCP type 1988/1989
* (W/100 m^3)

4.6   Among the factors which will result in an increased demand are buildings with greater depth, which will require higher standards of lighting and mechanical ventilation, much of which will be required to operate continuously.

4.7   Reservations in design should be made for the later introduction of known developments which may result in a substantial increase in demand for electrical power, for example, the application of food cook-chill facilities or a retro-fit of air-conditioning cooling method (from water cooling towers to forced-air cooling towers).

5.0 Supply voltage

5.1   The voltage at which the REC will deliver the supply will be determined by the facilities which can be made available, the prospective load and the extent of the HCP distribution system. The three options are:

a.   a low voltage (LV) supply (normally 240 V/415 V, 50 Hz, single or three phase, four wire) from the REC's LV network;

b.   a low voltage supply from a high voltage transformer sub-station located on a HCP property, which may be for the sole use of the HCP, or may jointly supply other consumers. This type of supply is suitable for medium-sized HCPs up to 500 kVA demand. The high voltage transformer and switchgear will remain the property of the REC;

c.   a high voltage (HV) supply (usually 11 kV three phase three wire) from the supply company's high voltage network. The HCP will be responsible for providing, operating and maintaining the high voltage transformers, associated switchgear and cabling on the consumer's side of the supply terminals (that is, after the metering equipment). The installation of a dedicated HV supply may be very expensive, but it may be easier for the supplier to offer the HCP an alternative, secure supply in the event of system load shedding. Consultation with the REC will be necessary at an early stage to ensure that a secure supply facility can be made available for the expected load at economically advantageous terms;

d.   in urban areas where the maximum demand of the HCP is large, the supply company may be able to provide a second HV feeder. Because of the interconnected nature of 11 kV supply networks, the increase in reliability which can be expected from a second feeder may be limited. In rural areas the additional cost of a second feeder may only be technically and economically advantageous for a large HCP where suitable overhead line and/or buried cable routes are available.

6.0 Diversity factors

6.1   Diversity can be allowed when calculating the size of main and sub-main circuit conductors and switchgear. The margin of diversity to be allowed requires a designer with special knowledge and experience, and must be applied to each particular installation individually. The whole HCP must be considered, taking into account future extensions as far as possible. The electrical power diversity factors applicable should be decided by the engineer responsible for design.

6.2   As a general guide, the following are diversity factors given in the IEE Wiring Regulations for a "current-rated" cable.

a.   lighting – 75% of total current;

b.   socket-outlets – 100% of largest load plus 50% of load demand in all other circuits;

c.   fixed equipment – 100% of largest load plus 75% of next largest load plus 40% of the remainder.

7.0 Distribution system

General concept

7.1   The distribution system should be designed to provide as much security of supply and flexibility for operation and safe maintenance as is possible within the cost limit allowance. Provision should be made in the design for any known future extensions. Adequate spare capacity should be allowed on bus-bars at main and sub-main feeders. Space should also be allowed for additional switching devices and distribution equipment, for example unequipped housings or bus-bar extension. The choice and type of distribution will be largely influenced by the size, shape, location and load centre of the premises.

7.2   At an early stage in the design, the distribution system should be assessed for operational requirements, fault levels, protection tripping times, and emergency supply provisions (see HTM 2011 – 'Emergency electrical services').

Essential services supply

7.3   The increasing dependence of medical and nursing procedures on electrical equipment calls for special attention to the electrical distribution system. Generating plant should be available to provide electrical power to those areas which will enable the HCP to carry out its essential functions. Within this general objective, the aim should be to simplify the electrical installations as far as practicable and avoid unnecessary segregation and repetition in essential and non-essential circuits, particularly for lighting circuits where comparatively small loads are involved.

7.4   Where new HCPs are built in separate construction phases the essential power supply for the whole should, as far as is possible, be planned and evaluated at the design stage. This will enable the total emergency power supply to be assessed in the early planning stages and appropriate areas of accommodation allocated. A.C. generator sets, as required, should be installed early in each of the phases of a development to ensure that the maximum security of emergency power is available at the outset and suitable staff training is obtained.

7.5   The essential power supply facilities for existing HCP should be periodically re-assessed and upgraded to ensure that sufficient emergency power supplies will always be connected to maintain essential clinical and surgical life-support facilities.

7.6   The connection of small or large electrical equipment to a supply system without regard to the current capacity of the installed cable and switching devices must be regulated. All fixed or portable items of electrical equipment which are expected to draw electrical power from the supply should be subject to registration for approved use by the authorised person. The on-cost of any new service, resulting in an increase of electrical power which exceeds the equipment or cable rated current/volt drop criteria, should include the additional electrical installation retro-fit costs necessary to ensure safety and reliability of operation.

7.7   The electrical distribution system should be simple, interlocked, safe, reliable and easy to maintain particularly where an 11 kV supply is envisaged (see HTM 2021 – 'Electrical safety code for high voltage systems' and HTM 2020 – 'Electrical safety code for low voltage systems').

7.8 Due to the larger increase in essential electrical supplies in proportion to non-essential supplies, it may be desirable that the essential and non-essential supply systems are combined into a single unified distribution system which is more economically advantageous than two segregated supply systems (see HTM 2011 – 'Emergency electrical services').

Cost parameters and present worth

7.9 The total cost of alternative distribution systems should be calculated for each particular project using the present worth technique of cost calculation. Present worth techniques are demonstrated in DoH documents ENG.D CE3.1/27 and ENG.D. CE6.1/33. The cost comparison should include:

    a. annual capital cost of electrical equipment and building spaces, based on a useful life of 30 years;

    b. annual cost of cable and transformer heat losses, where appropriate, allowing a load factor of 60% and based on the assumption that the most economic current rated cable is installed with a voltage drop of less than 4.0%;

    c. annual maintenance cost of electrical equipment;

    d. safety systems;

    e. cost of safety at work requirements of statutory regulations;

    f. cost of specialised staff and training requirements.

Ring or radial systems

7.10 The distribution circuits between the main incomer and load centres can be radial or ring distribution feeders. They should be designed to allow flexibility in operation and security of supply.

Maintenance of voltage

7.11 To comply with the IEE Wiring Regulations, low voltage installation circuit conductors should each have a voltage drop that does not exceed 4.0% from the supply terminals to the fixed current-using equipment at the full load current, disregarding motor starting conditions.

7.12 Where the supply from the REC is at high voltage, the HCP will generally be responsible for the operation of the complete installation including high voltage switchgear, cables and transformer(s).

7.13 Where two or more 11 kV feeders supply an HCP, the operation of these feeder circuit breakers will remain under the control of the REC. The REC will define the "supply terminals" at the point where the energy input is measured. This point will normally be near to the point of common coupling with the REC, at the 11 kV input to the transformer. The supply voltage will be subject to a statutory and limited variation of ±6% of the guaranteed LV at the main distribution switchboard.

7.14 A maximum cumulative 4.0% voltage drop from the main distribution switchboard to the fixed current-using equipment may result in a greater cable conductor area and overall diameter requirement, with increased purchase and installation cost.

7.15   To offset additional costs, the HCP main intake cables interconnecting the main distribution switchboard to the sub-main distribution switchboards should include, where the cable route length is significant, an additional voltage drop up to 3% maximum. This additional voltage drop (above the 4%) from the "supply terminals" to the "fixed-current using equipment" is subtracted from the ±6% voltage statutory variation allowed to the REC (Figure 2 refers). The estimated voltage drops should be calculated before deciding whether to use high voltage or low voltage for the main distribution. It may be found that low voltage systems are neither economic nor practicable due to unacceptable voltage drops or the additional cross-sectional area of cable required to comply with the IEE Wiring Regulations and the volume of the building space such cables would occupy.

7.16   The choice of the voltage for the main distribution will generally depend upon the economic considerations arising from the distances between the various load centres of the HCP and the main intake position. In marginal instances, preference should be given to high voltage for the main distribution system, for the reasons stated above. Where high voltage distribution is economically advantageous, 11 kV is the preferred voltage.

8.0 Abbreviations, staff functions and definitions

Abbreviations

8.1 Full forms of these are given below:

BS – British Standards issued by the British Standards Institution;

ERA – Electrical Research Association;

epr – ethylene propylene rubber complying with BS6899:1991;

hrc – high rupturing capacity;

ESI Std – Electricity Supply Industry Standard;

HV – high voltage (see "Definitions");

idmt – inverse definite minimum time;

IEE Wiring Regulations – Regulations for Electrical Installations issued by the Institution of Electrical Engineers (BS7671:1992 'The Requirements for Wiring Installations');

kA – kiloampere;

kV – kilovolt;

kVA – kilovolt-ampere;

kVAr – kilovolt-ampere, reactive;

kW – kilowatt;

LV – low voltage (see "Definitions");

MCB – miniature circuit breaker complying with BS3871 Part 1:1965 (1984);

MCCB – moulded case circuit breaker complying with BS EN 60947-2:1992;

mims – mineral insulated, metal sheathed;

mpfe – maximum prospective fault energy under symmetrical fault conditions, that is, a short circuit between all three phases;

mpfc – maximum prospective fault current;

MVA – megavolt-ampere;

pf – power factor;

pvc – polyvinyl chloride compound;

RCD – residual current device;

sir – silicon insulated rubber;

SF_6 – sulphur hexafluoride;

tlf – time limited fuses;

xlpe – cross-linked polyethylene compound.

Staff functions

8.2   Only trained, authorised and competent persons should be appointed by management to control the operation of electrical services.

8.3   Management: the owner, occupier, employer, general manager, chief executive or other person who is accountable for the premises and who is responsible for issuing or implementing a general policy statement under the HSW Act 1974.

Health and Safety at Work (Northern Ireland Order 1978 SI 1979/1039 NI9)

8.4   Designated person: an individual who has overall authority and responsibility for the premises containing the electrical supply and distribution system within the premises, and who has a duty under the HSW Act 1974 to prepare and issue a general policy statement on health and safety at work, including the organisation and arrangements for carrying out that policy. This person should not be the authorising engineer.

8.5   Duty holder: a person on whom the Electricity at Work Regulations 1989 impose a duty in connection with safety.

8.6   Employer: any person or body who:

a.   employs one or more individuals under a contract of employment or apprenticeship;

b   provides training under the schemes to which the Health and Safety (Training for Employment) Regulations 1988 (Statutory Instrument No 1988/1222) apply.

Northern Ireland: Health and Safety (Training for Employment) Regulations 1990, Statutory Instrument No 1990/1380

8.7   Authorising engineer (high voltage): a Chartered Electrical Engineer with appropriate experience and possessing the necessary degree of independence from local management, who is appointed in writing by management to implement, administer and monitor the safety arrangements for the high voltage electrical supply and distribution systems of that organisation to ensure compliance with the Electricity at Work Regulations 1989, and to assess the suitability and appointment of candidates in writing to be authorised persons (see HTM 2021 – 'Electrical safety code for high voltage systems').

8.8   Authorising engineer (low voltage): a Chartered Engineer or Incorporated Electrical Engineer with appropriate experience and possessing the necessary degree of independence from local management, who is appointed in writing by management to implement, administer and monitor the safety arrangements for the low voltage electrical supply and distribution systems of that organisation to ensure compliance with the Electricity at Work Regulations 1989, and to assess the suitability and appointment of candidates in writing to be authorised persons (see HTM 2020 – 'Electrical safety code for low voltage systems').

8.9   Authorised person: an individual possessing adequate technical knowledge and having received appropriate training, appointed in writing by the authorising engineer to be responsible for the practical implementation and operation of the management's safety policy and procedures on defined electrical systems (see HTMs 2020 and 2021).

8.10   Competent person: an individual who, in the opinion of an Authorised Person, has sufficient technical knowledge and experience to prevent danger while carrying out work on defined electrical systems (see HTMs 2020 and HTM 2021).

The suffix "electrical" associated with the definitions "authorised person" and "competent person" will only be used with letters of appointment to provide a clear differentiation between persons having similar titles but appointed for different duties, that is, medical gas systems, etc. The suffix has not been included against these terms when used within this document but is, however, implicit.

Definitions

8.11   Department: an abbreviation of the generic term "UK Health Departments" (the Department of Health, the Scottish Office, the Welsh Office and the Department of Health and Social Services Northern Ireland).

8.12   Injury: death or personal injury from electrical shock, electrical burn, electrical explosion or arcing, or from fire or explosion initiated by electrical energy.

8.13   Danger: a risk of injury.

8.14   System: a system in which all the electrical equipment is, or may be, electrically connected to a common source of electrical energy, including such source and such equipment.

8.15   Essential circuits: circuits forming part of the essential services electrical supply, so arranged that they can be supplied separately from the remainder of the electrical installation.

8.16   Generator set: an engine-driven synchronous a.c. generator with exciter and other essential components to generate electrical power, that is, which can be started and run independently of any external electrical supply.

8.17   Emergency supply: any form of electrical supply which is intended to be available in the event of a failure in the normal supply.

8.18   Essential service electrical supply: the supply from an engine-driven a.c. emergency generator which is arranged to come into operation in the event of a failure of the normal supply and provide sufficient electrical energy to ensure that all basic functions of the HCP are maintained in service.

8.19   No-break supply: a circuit continuously energised whether or not the normal supply is available.

8.20   Electrical equipment: includes anything used, intended to be used or installed for use to generate, provide, transmit, transform, conduct, distribute, control, measure or use electrical energy.

8.21   Equipment: abbreviation of electrical equipment.

8.22   High voltage (HV): the existence of a potential difference (rms value for a.c.) normally exceeding 1000 volts a.c. between circuit conductors, or 600 volts between circuit conductors and earth.

8.23   Low voltage (LV): the existence of a potential difference (rms value for a.c.) not exceeding 1000 volts a.c. or 1500 volts d.c. between circuit conductors, or 600 volts a.c. or 900 volts d.c. between circuit conductors and earth.

8.24   Conductor: a conductor of electrical energy.

8.25   Circuit conductor: any conductor in a system which is intended to carry electrical current in normal conditions, but does not include a conductor provided solely to perform a protective function by connection to earth or other reference point.

8.26   Connected equipment: equipment connected into the low voltage system utilising electrical power to perform its dedicated function.

8.27   Discrimination: means by which protective devices separate faulty equipment from sound. Discrimination exists where the protection is so graded that when a fault occurs, only the protective device nearest to, and upstream from, the point of fault operates.

8.28   Load factor: the ratio of the number of electrical units supplied during a given period to the number that would have been supplied had the maximum demand been maintained throughout the period: usually expressed as a percentage.

8.29   Space factor: the ratio (expressed as a percentage) of the total cross-sectional area of bunched cables including insulation, sleeving and armouring divided by the internal cross-sectional area of the conduit, duct, trunking, etc in which the cables are installed.

8.30   Flame retardant: cable with a cover and an insulation which inhibits continuity of combustion and will not cause the fire to spread. The cable will not support combustion 60 seconds after removal of heat source. Tested to BS4066:Part 1:1980.

8.31   Fire-resistant: cable which will continue to operate during a fire. Tested to BS6387:1983 (1991) and graded for a specific temperature range.

8.32   Reduced flame: cable designed to meet stringent requirements for limiting flame propagation when bunched.

8.33   Low smoke: cable with halogen-free compounds and low smoke characteristics in a fire.

8.34   Residual current: the vector sum of the instantaneous values of current flowing through all live conductors of a circuit at a point in the electrical installation (IEE Wiring Regulations).

8.35   Residual current device: a mechanical switching device or association of devices intended to cause the opening of the contacts when the residual current attains a given value under specified conditions (IEE Wiring Regulations).

9.0 References

British Standards Institution (Specifications):

The degree of correspondence between IEC, ISO and BSI standards is indicated by the following symbols:

≡   a standard identical in every detail;

=   a technically equivalent standard with different presentation;

≠   related, but not equivalent standard.

BS31:1940 (1988) Steel conduits and fittings for electrical wiring.

BS88 Cartridge fuses, for voltages up to and including 1000 V a.c. and 1500 V d.c. – General requirements. (≡ IEC 269–1)

BS88:Part 2 Fuses for use by authorised persons. (mainly for industrial applications)

BS88:Section 2.1:1988 Supplementary requirements. (≡ IEC 269–2)

BS89:Part 1:1990 Single purpose direct acting electrical indicating instruments and their accessories. Definitions and general requirements common to all parts. (≡ EN 60 051–1, IEC 51–1)

BS159:1992 High voltage bus-bars and bus-bar connections.

BS171 Power transformers. Parts 1, 2, 3, 4 and 5.

BS697:1977 Rubber gloves for electrical purposes.

BS921:1976 (1987) Rubber mats for electrical purposes.

BS1361:1971 (1986) Cartridge fuses for a.c. circuits in domestic and similar premises. (≠ IEC269–1)

BS1362:1973 (1992) General purpose fuse links for domestic and similar puposes. (primarily for use in plugs) (≠ IEC269–1)

BS1363:1984 13A fused plugs and switched and unswitched socket-outlets.

BS1387:1985 (1990) Steel tubes and tubulars suitable for welding or screwing to BS21 pipe threads. (= ISO65)

BS1650:1971 Capacitors for connection to power-frequency systems. (= IEC70)

BS2484:1985 Straight concrete and clayware cable covers.

BS2692:Part 1:1986 Current-limiting fuses. (≡ IEC282–1)

BS2757:1986 Method for determining the thermal classification of electrical insulation. (≡ IEC85)

BS2870:1980 Rolled copper and copper alloys. Sheet, strip and foil.

BS2874:1986 Copper and copper alloys. Rods and sections (other than forging stock).

BS2898:1970 (1985) Wrought aluminium and aluminium alloys for electrical purposes. Bars, extruded round tube and sections.

BS3535:Parts 1 & 2:1990 Isolating transformers and safety isolating transformers. (Part 1, ≡ EN 60 742)

BS3871:Part 1:1965 (1984) Miniature air-break circuit-breakers for a.c. circuits. (≠ IEC898)

BS3938:1973 (1992) Current transformers. (≠ IEC185)

BS4066:Part 1:1980 Method of test on a single vertical insulated wire or cable. (≡ IEC332–1)

BS4196:Part 0:1981 (1986) Guide for the use of basic standards and for the preparation of noise test codes. (≡ ISO 374)

BS4293:1983 Residual current-operated circuit-breakers. (≠ IEC755)

BS4568:Part 1:1970 Steel conduit, bends and couplers. (≠ CEE23)

BS4568:Part 2:1970 (1988) Fittings and components. (≠ CEE23)

BS4752: Switchgear and controlgear for voltages up to and including 1000 volts a.c. and 1200 volts d.c. Part 1: 1977 (1990) Circuit breakers. (≠ IEC157–1, IEC157–1A, IEC157–1B)

BS5045 All parts: Transportable gas containers.

BS5227:1992 A.c. metal-enclosed switchgear and controlgear for rated voltages above 1 kV and up to and including 52 kV. (≠ IEC298)

BS5463: High-voltage switches. Part 2 (1991) High-voltage switches for rated voltages of 52 kV and above. (≡ IEC265–2: 1988)

BS5467:1989 Cables with thermosetting insulation for electricity supply for rated voltages up to and including 600/1000 V and up to and including 1900/3300 V. (≠ IEC502, IEC811)

BS5486 Low-voltage switchgear and controlgear assemblies. Part 1: 1990 Requirements for type-tested and partially type-tested assemblies. (≡ EN 60 439–1, ≠ IEC439–1)

BS5685 Electricity meters. Part 1: 1979 (1992). (= IEC521); Part 3: 1986 (1992). (≠ IEC211)

BS6004:1991 Pvc-insulated cables (non-armoured) for electric power and lighting. (≠ IEC227)

BS6007:1991 Rubber-insulated cables for electric power and lighting. (≠ IEC245)

BS6121 Mechanical cable glands (all parts).

BS6207:Part 1:1991 Mineral-insulated copper-sheathed cables with copper conductors. (≠ IEC702–1: 1988)

BS6346:1989 Pvc-insulated cables for electricity supply.

BS6387:1983 (1991) Performance requirements for cables required to maintain circuit integrity under fire conditions.

BS6480:1988 Impregnated paper-insulated lead or lead alloy sheathed electric cables of rated voltage up to and including 33,000 V. (≠ IEC55–1, IEC55–2)

BS6500:1990 Insulated flexible cords and cables. (≠ IEC227, IEC245)

BS6581:1985 (1992) Common requirements for high-voltage switchgear and controlgear standards. (≠ IEC694:1980)

BS6622:1991 Cables with extruded/cross-linked polyethylene or ethylene propylene rubber insulation for rated voltages from 3800/6600 V up to to 19,000/33,000 V.

BS6724:1990 Armoured cables for electricity supply having thermosetting insulation with low emission of smoke and corrosive gases when affected by fire.

BS6899:1991 Rubber insulation and sheath of electric cables.

BS7671:1992 The requirements for wiring installations (the IEE Wiring Regulations 16th edition).

British Standards Institution (Codes of Practice):

BS6423:1983 Maintenance of electrical switchgear and controlgear for voltages up to and including 650 V.

BS6651:1985 Protection of structures against lightning.

BS7430:1991 Earthing.

CP1010:1975 Loading guide of oil immersed transformers. (≠ IEC694:1980)

Electricity Association:

EA Standards and Engineering recommendations:

35–1:1985 Distribution transformers (from 16 kVA to 1000 kVA)

41–26:1991 Distribution switchgear. Ratings up to 36 kV.

C89.1:1986 Termination on polymeric insulation cables rated at 12 kV and 36 kV.

G59:1985 Connection of private generating plant at the electricity supply system.

ET113:1989 Guidance for the protection of private generating sets up to 5 MW, in parallel with the Regional Electricity Company distribution network.

G5/3 (1976) Limits for harmonics in the UK electricity supply system.

Electrical Research Association:

ERA 69–30 Part III Sustained current ratings for pvc-insulated cables. Part 5, Sustained current ratings for cables with thermosetting insulation.

American National Standards Inst & Inst of Electrical and Electronic Engineers:

ANSI/IEEE C62.41:1980 Surge voltages in low voltage a.c. power circuits.

10.0 Symbols used in diagrams
(as recommended by BS1192:Part 3, 1987)

⅄	Socket-outlet
⊗	Indicator lamp
	Switch or isolator
	Isolator used as bus-section switch
	Manually operated changeover switch
	Fuse link
	Fuse
	Fuse switch
	Circuit breaker
	Contactor
	Electric motor starter
	Changeover contactor comprising two contactors with mechanical and electrical interlocks
	Relay or contactor operating coil
	Push-button switch
	Self-contained escape/standby luminaire
	Double wound transformer
	Storage battery
	Horn or hooter
Ⓖ	Synchronous AC generator
	Control panel
avr	Automatic voltage regulator
	Connection to earth conductor or earth electrode.

11.0 Distribution and cable systems

High voltage distribution

General

11.1　Where high voltage is employed for the main distribution system, the aim should be to cover as much of the network as is practicable with high voltage (HV) cables and keep the low voltage (LV) cables as short as possible. The system should be simple, consistent with safety, and offer a degree of discrimination under fault conditions which will limit disconnections to a minimum. Systems of various connections to the regional electricity company (REC) are shown in Figure 5.

11.2　Arrangements should be made to trip the high voltage intake switchgear, which is owned and controlled by the REC, in an emergency. A safe and secure point of access and retreat should be provided for personnel for this operation. HCP transformers and sub-stations should always be fed from HV switchgear which is under the control of the management. Switchgear should be duplicated, if necessary, as shown in Figure 5.

11.3　All electrical equipment and cable works must be capable of dealing safely with the maximum prospective fault current (mpfc) to which it is subjected by the supply system. The fault level at the HCP supply intake will depend upon the arrangement of the supply authority's distribution network, and the most onerous value should be obtained from the supply authority. High voltage distribution equipment, which forms part of the HCP installation, should be arranged to minimise the LV fault level. This is achieved by limiting the rating of transformers and providing interlocks on bus-bar couplers to prevent paralleling of supply feeders and transformers. Advice on fault current calculations is given in BS5311:1988 and BS4752 (see section 20).

11.4　High voltage system protection should limit the extent of supply interruptions under fault conditions, considered in conjunction with the provision of emergency supplies generating capacity (see HTM 2011 – 'Emergency electrical services') which is provided to maintain essential services during interruptions of the normal supply.

Ring or radial distribution

11.5　The distribution circuits between the main intake and load centres may be radial or ring distribution feeders, and should be designed to allow flexibility and security of supply:

  a.　ring distribution:

    (i)　high voltage, fused-switch protected, ring main units used for distribution transformers connected to a ring distribution system, would generally provide a satisfactory arrangement (see Figure 3). This system would normally operate as an open ring so that a fault on one leg of the ring would cause a loss of supply in that leg only. The probability of a fault on the HV distribution system is small, making this a generally secure arrangement, particularly where automatic standby generator(s) are available for supplying any LV essential circuits during loss of normal supply;

(ii) it is unlikely that a higher degree of tripping selectivity will be required, but where this can be justified, the design and commissioning should only be undertaken by protection experts;

b. radial distribution:

(i) with radial distribution, isolation of a fault is limited to the faulty section only. To provide some of the flexibility for maintenance inherent in a ring distribution system, it is desirable to provide the low voltage interconnectors shown in Figure 7 which are typical of a radial distribution system. The emergency supplies are not shown, these being in accordance with HTM 2011 – 'Emergency electrical services'.

11.6   An alternative emergency supply distribution system, which is not specifically referred to in HTM 2011 – 'Emergency electrical services', is shown in Figure 8, the normal supplies being HV radial feeders and the emergency supply system being an LV ring main system. With a single generator system the LV ring main would normally operate closed. The ring main would operate open if two unsynchronised generators were used.

Circuit protection

11.7   Figure 19 shows typical main distribution protection that is used in HCPs to give adequate discrimination. It will be clear from Figures 3, 4 and 9 that the principles are applicable to both ring or radial HV main distribution systems. Where a transformer supplies only one local switchboard it may be necessary to provide, in addition to HV overcurrent protection, an earth fault intertrip circuit protection at the LV earth connection and overcurrent protection at the LV circuit breaker of the 415 V switchboard. Ring main compact distribution transformers will be provided with either HV fuse links or current transformer operated switch protection.

Low voltage distribution

General

11.8   All distribution equipment, that is, switching devices, fuse boards, bus-bars, cables and wiring, should be fully rated for the estimated maximum loading with spare capacity based on foreseeable future growth. Special attention should be given to balance the loads between phases.

11.9   Circuit breakers, fuse-switches and bus-bars should be rated to handle safely the mpfc of the system. Where the supply is obtained from a high voltage transformer having a capacity of 500 kVA, or less, the mpfc of the main low voltage system may generally be within the limits of circuit breakers of 20 kA rating. A 1000 kVA transformer will probably need circuit breakers rated at 50 kA. Where an HCP has HV or LV generating plant operating in parallel with the main supplies, the mpfc of the HCP system should be evaluated for the worst case.

11.10   The type of distribution used will be influenced largely by the layout of the HCP and location of large loads. Continuity of supply is particularly important, and where economically practicable, use of interconnectors or ring circuits should be considered to enable the supply to be maintained in the event of a fault involving a major component.

11.11   A line diagram of a typical low voltage radial distribution system is shown in Figure 10.

Cable ratings

11.12   Except in special circumstances, for example circuits for fixed X-ray equipment, it is important that the maximum voltage drop complies with the requirements of the IEE Wiring Regulations. The current ratings of conductors are given in the tables of the IEE Wiring Regulations and IEC publication 287: 'Calculation of continuous current ratings of cables'. The appropriate cable conductor rating factor for current limiting protection devices may be applied where ratings are quoted for back-up overcurrent protection (see paragraphs 11.14 and 11.15).

11.13   The voltage drop can be readily calculated from the conductor current rating tables included in the IEE Wiring Regulations or manufacturer's brochures, using the data appropriate for the type of cable.

Circuit protection

11.14   Special attention should be given to the protection of electrical circuits in HCPs due to the increasing dependence upon the use of electrical equipment. The rapid isolation of faulty circuits without affecting healthy ones can be achieved by the use of protection devices, for example enclosed current limiting fuse links complying with BS88:Part 1; and miniature circuit breakers (MCBs) complying with BS3871:Part 1. Moulded case circuit breakers (MCCBs) complying with BS4752 are recommended for larger industrial applications of electrical current. Semi-enclosed rewireable fuses should no longer be used.

11.15   Where equipment is supplied with electrical power, protection should be provided. This would ensure that, under fault conditions, the equipment would be disconnected before thermal effects damage it and/or the cabling beyond repair. Protection should therefore be provided for overload conditions and for maximum prospective fault currents. Figures 18 and 19 show how discrimination may be achieved using overcurrent protection of the type specified above. The graphs are only typical of some of the many curves available for fuse links, MCBs and MCCBs, and are intended to demonstrate how discrimination may be calculated and planned.

Miniature circuit breakers, moulded case circuit breakers and fuse links

11.16   MCBs are available in current ratings up to 100 A, and MCCBs in current ratings up to 5000 A in the fixed pattern and up to 2500 A in the draw-out pattern. It can be seen from Table 2 that the fault current handling capacities of MCBs and MCCBs are not time extended to the same degree as a fuse link. The fuse link is wholly a thermal device, whereas the MCB and MCCB are both combined thermal and magnetic devices. The magnetic device gives an instantaneous cutoff to the current-time inverse characteristic curve, at a set gate value of current and time, not in excess of 0.1 second. In the system example shown in Figure 19 and Table 10, a class M1 MCB, that is an MCB of 1 kA rated fault current capacity, would not be suitable for the 100 A unit because it is not rated to pass the 1.5 kA prospective fault current at point 2, and is at the extreme rating of load currents for MCBs. In such a situation it would be necessary to choose a switching device of higher rating and fault current capacity.

Rated current "In" for gG or gM fuses (A)	BS88:Parts 1/5/6/2 1988 (1992)			MCBs – BS3871:Part1 1965 (1984) MCCBs – BS4752		
	Conventional time (hours)	Conventional current (A)		Category of duty	Current rating (A)	Short circuit (kA)
		Inf	If			
				MCBs:		
				M 4.5	6–50	4.5
In–16	1			M 6	6–63	6.0
16–63	1	1.25In	1.6In	M9	6–63	9.0
				MCCBs.	10–100	8.0
63–160	2				25–200	25.0
160–400	3				125–250	20.0
400–In	4				250–400	25.0

Table 2   Comparative fault current handling capacity of current limiting gG and gM fuse links, MCBs and MCCBs

Inf = non-fusing current. If = fusing current. In = nominal rated current

11.17   In phase-to-earth faults, the fault current is limited to the quotient of the phase voltage and the earth fault loop impedance. In phase-to-phase faults the current is limited to the quotient of the line voltage and the circuit impedance of the two or three phases. Care must be exercised in selecting an upstream MCCB to discriminate for a large through fault current.

11.18   With a downstream MCB, especially in single phase circuits, MCCB and MCB characteristic curves converge for fault currents at approximately 10 milliseconds, thus losing discrimination in the MCB circuit; this is defined as partial discrimination. The simple solution is to use an enclosed current limiting fuse (hrc) of suitable rating, that is, at 1.6 times the subcircuit's rating, to replace the MCCB. The fuse link and MCB curves cross over at the MCB minimum time. The fuse link curtails the time of any large fault current and limits circuit damage.

11.19   MCBs and fuse links are rated as suitable for a maximum continuous current. The non-adjustable instantaneous tripping levels of MCBs are based on multiples of the continuously rated current (In). There are four levels or types of MCB, set for designers by BS3871:Part 1: these are types 1, 2, 3 and 4. They are required to operate within 0.1 second at the instantaneous current limiting gate values:

Type 1 – between 2.7 In and 4 In
Type 2 – between 4.0 In and 7 In   These are non-adjustable instantaneous
Type 3 – between 7.0 In and 10 In   current limiting gate values.
Type 4 – between 10.0 In and 50 In

11.20   For indirect contact, it is an IEE Wiring Regulations requirement for TN-S systems that socket-outlets at 240 V used for portable apparatus must be disconnected in less than 0.4 second. At 415 V, 3-phase disconnection is reduced to less than 0.1 second. All fixed apparatus must be disconnected in less than 5.0 seconds. In earthed systems, the loop impedance of any connected electrical circuit must reflect the type number of the MCB used to satisfy, at worst, the requirement of 0.1 second, 0.4 second or 5.0 seconds to trip.

11.21   The earth fault loop impedance (phase-to-earth loop) may be defined as starting and ending at the point of earth fault. Within buildings this is basically understood to mean the impedance sums of the phase circuit conductor and the common parallel paths of the neutral, protective conductor and cable armour back to the point of supply at the transformer star point neutral. The value of the maximum fault current that can flow depends upon the earth fault loop impedance and the applied voltage. This will dictate the correct type number MCB at the required rated current, for example:

a.   voltage 240 V, earth fault loop impedance 2 ohms, appliance rating 10 A, MCB rating In = 16 amps. Maximum possible earth fault current = 240/2 = 120 A. Type 2 MCB – (4 In–7 In) – gate value to operate instantaneously between 64 A and 112 A, within 0.1 second, would be suitable;

b.   types 3 and 4 would not operate instantaneously at the above earth current; however, they would operate in slower time along the thermal inverse time characteristic curve. This would not satisfy the 0.4 second disconnection requirement, but might still be suitable for the 5.0 second trip requirement for a fixed appliance.

11.22   At all times the in-rush starting load current to equipment must be known. This applies in particular to transformers, motors, tungsten or discharge lighting. Care must be exercised to ensure that the MCB does not trip on start-up.

11.23   Cable continuous ratings must always be greater than the current rating of the protective devices, and exceed the time interval required for the protection to operate to prevent cable thermal damage during equipment overload. Fuses specified in BS88:Part 1 (IEC296-1:1986) have been allocated a "breaking range" and a "utilisation category". The "breaking range" is indicated by the first letter, lower case "a" or "g", and the "utilisation category" by the second letter, upper case "G" or "M", as follows:

a.   "g" fuse links – (full range breaking capacity);

b.   "a" fuse links – (partial-range breaking capacity);

c.   "G" – indicates general circuit protection;

d.   "M" – indicates motor circuit protection.

The fusing current (If) capacity of "gG" and "gM" fuse links is shown in Table 2.

11.24   Both the inverse time delay (thermal) and instantaneous overcurrent release protection settings of an MCCB are adjustable within a limited range. For current settings greater than 63 A, thermal tripping from a cold state will not occur in less than 2 hours. This can vary between 1.05 and 1.25 times current setting.

11.25   Instantaneous current operation will be activated within ±10% of its overload current setting (BS4752 refers). The MCB, which is non-adjustable, can be chosen with types 1, 2, 3, or 4 instantaneous current limiting gate values.

11.26   The fault breaking current capacity range of the MCCB is 8 kA to 50 kA.

Residual current devices

11.27   "Residual current device" (RCD) is a generic term to describe several types of insulation protective devices which continuously monitor the insulation resistance of an electrical circuit. Failure in the insulation material or direct contact by personnel could activate the device. The RCD senses difference in the values of the circuit current flowing in the live and neutral wires. The imbalance in current is usually set at 300, 100, 30 or 10 milliamperes with operating times of 40 or 200 milliseconds. A summary of operating qualities is shown in Table 3.

	RCDs		
	RCCB Residual current circuit breaker	RCBO Residual current circuit breaker	RCD relays control relay
Isolation	T	O	D
Switching	T	T	D
Volt free control contacts			T
Earth fault protection	T	T	T
Overload protection		T	D
Discriminatory time delay	O		O
Phase/neutral switching	T	T	D

T – typical features
O – optional features
D – dependent on main circuit breaker
Table 3

11.28 Groups of items of equipment with a total earth leakage current in excess of 50% of the circuit RCD set operating current should not be connected to the same circuit outlet. Failure to observe this requirement may result in spurious trip operation of the RCD. Several steps to trouble-free operation with RCDs are to select:

a. RCD with filter;

b. RCD or RCBO (combined MCB/RCD, IEC 1009);

c. RCD with shortest operating time nearest the load;

d. RCD upstream time-delayed;

e. circuit grouping to avoid total excessive earth leakage current;

f. power factor corrected light fittings;

or to avoid the use of mims cable with large total capacitance.

11.29 When to use an RCD:

a. where the earth fault loop impedance is too high for rapid automatic disconnection by the circuit protective device;

b. on circuits supplying socket-outlets which are outside the equipotential protected zone;

c. on TT circuits;

d. in laboratories and workshops;

e. in equipment supplied by trailing leads;

f. in fire prevention, as a means of detecting and isolating a cable, or electrical equipment of high impedance earth fault leakage current.

Fixed X-ray equipment circuits

11.30 The special feature of circuits for X-ray apparatus is the transient nature of the loads. This feature can cause interference with other parts of the installation. To reduce this effect, circuits supplying permanently connected X-ray equipment should be taken from separate sub-main feeders. Though comparatively heavy currents are used, the duration of the peak load rarely exceeds 1 second. There is therefore no problem of excess temperature rise, but it is important that the circuit wiring should be capable of carrying the maximum load without undue voltage drop. A maximum permissible voltage drop or source impedance is usually specified by the makers of X-ray equipment. The sizes of the circuit conductors should be chosen to satisfy these requirements. Voltage drop has to be given at a known current; a typical value is 5% voltage drop.

11.31   Because of the transient loading of X-ray circuits, considerable diversity factors can be allowed in determining the sizes of circuit wiring when several machines are supplied from the same sub-main board. A diversity factor can also be allowed in determining the rating of distribution switchgear supplying X-ray circuits because the switchgear is never likely to be required to make or break the circuit under peak load conditions. Suggested diversity factors are:

a.   two machines – none;

b.   three machines – 100% largest load plus 50% other loads.

The use of ring circuits will usually achieve a considerable saving in conductor size and also assist in reducing voltage drop where more than two X-ray machines have to be supplied; socket-outlets for use with mobile X-ray circuits are dealt with in paragraph 11.32.

Mobile X-ray units

11.32   With regard to sub-circuits and socket-outlets used with mobile X-ray units:

a.   mobile X-ray machines should be supplied from standard general-purpose 13 amp socket-outlets preferably wired in a ring circuit. To ensure that the full rated output of mobile X-ray units is available during the exposure period, manufacturers recommend a maximum value for the supply impedance at any socket-outlet to which the unit may be connected;

b.   provided that the known current for a maximum volt drop requirement, which as stated in the IEE Wiring Regulations is 4.0% (that is, 9.6 V where the declared voltage is 240 V), is complied with, the total source impedance at any standard general-purpose socket-outlet can be expected to be less than 0.54 ohm. This is the maximum design value of source impedance that should be used;

c.   in addition to ensuring satisfactory voltage drop conditions it is necessary to ensure that the close current protection of the 13 amp socket-outlets will not operate under normal X-ray operating conditions, for example during the brief exposure period. The majority of modern mobile X-ray units have relatively low current requirements and use only their batteries or capacitor banks during the exposure period;

d.   these units should be fitted with fused 13 amp plugs and fuses complying with BS1363 (1984) and BS1362:1973 (1992) for the protection of the sub-circuit or socket-outlets. X-ray units (for example D38 model) having up to 300 mA rating, are fitted with 56/0.3 mm (4 mm^2) or 84/0.3 mm (6 mm^2) flexible cables and use special non-fused 13 amp plugs marked "X-ray". Current limiting fuses type aG complying with BS88 and thermal/magnetic MCBs type 3 are more suitable for the protection of 30 amp ring circuits when used for supplying these mobile X-ray units up to 300 mA exposure current. Types 1 and 2 of 30 amp magnetic/thermal MCBs, and some fuses, are too sensitive for this application as they are liable to operate during exposures to impulse current at the maximum rating of the X-ray units;

e. socket-outlets which are used extensively for the D38 X-ray units should be engraved "X-ray" and a small indelibly marked self-adhesive label should be attached to the socket-outlets to indicate the supply impedance to that point. Details of the measurement and marking of socket-outlets for these units are given in paragraph 11.33;

f. for satisfactory patient and operator safety, fixed or portable residual current devices (RCD), set at 30 mA, should be fitted.

Impedance measurement of socket-outlets used for mobile X-ray units

11.33   The following methods are used:

a. the impedance at socket-outlets which will be extensively used for mobile X-ray units up to 300 mA rating should be measured on completion of the installation, using a line-to-neutral impedance tester;

b. the total source impedance at any socket-outlet in an HCP having an installation which complies with the IEE Wiring Regulations can be expected to be less than 0.34 ohm, so the full rated output of the mobile X-ray unit will be available;

c. when using socket-outlets with lower source impedance it is necessary to add an impedance within the mobile X-ray unit to achieve a total circuit impedance of 0.34 ohm. The mobile X-ray unit impedance correction switch has steps for this purpose, each identified by a number;

d. socket-outlets which are used for mobile X-ray units should be identified with a number, from 1 to 6, using self-adhesive label or engraving, which indicates the mains impedance at that socket-outlet. Table 4 sets out the mains impedance and corresponding number.

Indicating number	Socket-outlet: line to neutral impedance (ohms)					
1	–	0.01	0.03	0.05	0.07	0.08
2	0.04	0.06	0.08	0.1	0.12	1.13
3	0.09	0.11	0.13	0.15	0.17	0.18
4	0.14	0.16	0.18	0.2	0.22	0.23
5	0.19	0.21	0.23	0.25	0.27	0.28
6	0.24	0.26	0.28	0.3	0.32	0.33
Mains volts*	200 V	210 V	220 V	230 V	250 V	250V

* Nominal mains voltage at "supply terminals"

Table 4   Number marking for socket-outlets extensively used for mobile X-ray units

Lift circuits

11.34   The essential service generation and load should be adequate to absorb any regenerative braking load requirement of the lift drive motors. Because of the fluctuating nature of the lift motor loads, they should be supplied from a separate essential services sub-main feeder.

11.35   Hydraulic lifts require a much greater input of power than is required for traction drive lifts. Hydraulic lifts are not normally used to service more than three floor levels.

11.36   Lifts with a variable speed control are of the traction drive type. The source of power is regulated by solid state devices. It is essential that this supply should be filtered at the equipment input to reduce the injection of harmonic voltages back into the supply mains or to the a.c. emergency generator. Electricity Association document G5/3 'Harmonics in the UK supply' refers.

11.37   The nominated fireman lift should be provided with a segregated essential supply. Emergency/fire escape bed lifts should be provided with two segregated cable routes from the essential supplies. Only cables for the operation of a particular lift may be routed in that lift shaft.

11.38   Lifts for use in HCPs should conform to all the relevant parts of BS5655: 'Lifts and service lifts', Health Technical Memorandum 2011 - 'Emergency electrical services' ("Design considerations") and NHS Model Engineering Specification C42 parts A, B and C.

Petrol filling stations

11.39   Health and Safety Executive document HS(G) 41 recommends that the electrical supply to petrol filling stations should not be connected to earth by means of a protective multi-earth system (TN-C-S). Earthing should only be by means of a system where the neutral and protective conductor are completely separate (TN-S). This should apply whether or not the petrol filling station forms an integral part of the HCP.

11.40   A test cabinet should be provided at the point of local supply for routine operational checks, which involve the connection of test instruments for measurement of the earth fault loop impedance and the RCD protection.

Internal low voltage distribution and utilisation circuits

General

11.41   As far as is reasonably practicable, the type of cable selected should be suitable for the ambient conditions in which it is to be installed, special attention being given to temperature, risk of mechanical damage, ease of installation and allowances for subsequent alterations and additions. Copper conductors are preferred in all cases.

11.42   Fire precautions are of special importance in all HCPs. Fire barriers and cable penetration seals are recommended along all cable routes. Fire-retardant, low-smoke, halogen-free cables are also recommended for use in all circuits which are located in, or pass through, spaces that would present a hazard to patients, staff, the general public and high value equipment. Reference should be made to the following Health Technical Memoranda:

> HTM 81 – 'Firecode: Fire precautions in new hospitals';
> HTM 82 – 'Firecode: Alarm and detection systems';
> HTM 83 – 'Fire safety in healthcare premises: general fire precautions';
> HTM 85 – 'Firecode: Fire precautions in existing hospitals';
> HTM 86 – 'Firecode: Fire risks assessment in existing hospitals;
> HTM 87 – 'Firecode: Textiles and furniture';
> HTM 88 – 'Fire safety in health care premises: Guide to fire precautions in NHS housing in the community for mentally handicapped/ill people'.

Electrical interference

11.43   Another important aspect is the need to minimise electromagnetic interference which will affect the use of sensitive medical electrical apparatus and data handling equipment. This demands that all cables and wiring in areas subject to interference should have a continuous metallic earth bonded screen and/or be enclosed in steel conduit, trunking or cabinets which are magnetically sealed, and electrically bonded to earth. Phase, neutral and protective conductors should also be installed within the same earthed and sealed enclosure.

11.44   Due to the need to minimise electrical interference, systems of wiring such as earthed sheath return wiring (esrw; TN-C) and protective multiple earthing (pme, or TN-C-S) must not be used in HCPs. With such systems, neutral currents may flow along the structural metalwork as a path to earth and cause induced magnetic fields. The abatement of electrical interference is dealt with more fully in HTM 2014 – 'Abatement of electrical interference'.

11.45   BS6667 Parts 1, 2, 3 – 'Electromagnetic compatibility for industrial process measurement and control equipment' refers. Various EN specifications supported by EC Directive 89/336/EEC will be legally enforceable.

11.46   In residential accommodation and areas where the domestic equipment is not sensitive to interference, normal domestic type wiring installations are satisfactory, for example non-armoured pvc conduit, insulated pvc sheathed wiring complying with BS6004, provided it is protected against the possibility of mechanical damage as required by the IEE Wiring Regulations.

Materials corrosion

Application of bitumen or bitumenised paint before assembly is an effective precaution against corrosion.

11.47   In damp situations, special precautions should be taken to prevent cable sheaths or armour, metal conduits, gland fittings and trunking systems from coming into contact with any of the following:

a.   materials containing magnesium chloride which are used in the construction of floors;

b.   plaster undercoats contaminated with corrosive salts;

c.   lime, cement and plaster, for example on unpainted walls;

d.   oak and other acidic woods;

e.   dissimilar metals liable to set up electrolytic action;

f.   acidic and humid atmospheres;

g.   polystyrene foam in contact with cable sheaths such as pvc;

h.   metal conduits laid in concrete, which is not certified as free of organic salts and/or aggressive additives.

Internal feeder cables

11.48   The grades of cable insulation normally used are pvc cables complying with BS6004, epr cables complying with BS6007 or xlpe cables complying with BS6234 and BS6622. Experience has shown that pvc insulated cables have superior mechanical properties, and are preferable for ambient temperature conditions within the range 0–65°C. They are therefore suitable for most HCP applications where a low-smoke, non-toxic, halogen-free, fire-resistant cable safety criterion is **not** required.

11.49   Both xlpe and epr insulated cables are suitable for ambient temperatures up to 80°C. Cables with xlpe outer sleeves and bedding can be laid in temperatures down to minus 40°C. When pvc outer sleeves are used the minimum laying temperature is as for pvc insulated cables, that is, temperatures above 0°C.

11.50   Non-armoured silicon rubber insulated cables complying with BS6007 are suitable for use in temperatures up to 145°C. General application of silicon rubber insulated cables will be rare, because fire-resistant cables to BS6387 will usually be preferred in high ambient temperatures.

11.51   Fire-retardant pvc, xlpe and epr or fire-resistant cables are suitable for internal feeders. The recommendations for low voltage distribution cables (see paragraph 16.34) apply equally for external and internal distribution. The cable outer sheaths and bedding should preferably be of non-toxic, halogen-free gas emitting compound/material. This is dependent upon the operational sensitivity and the safety criteria required under fire conditions.

11.52   Fire-retardant cables subjected to heat will burn freely when assembled in a large mass. The installation should conform to BS4066:Part 3, or IEC332:Part 3 – 'Flame characteristics of bunched cable installations'.

11.53   At intersections and junctions of routes, cables should be labelled and identified with permanent labels.

11.54   Each penetration of a structural fire barrier by any cable traywork or trunking system should be fully sealed with approved fire-resistant barrier material. Where extensive fire barrier material is required, the cable rating may need re-assessment. Appropriate cable current ratings, and voltage drop values can be found in the manufacturer's literature.

11.55   All bare wire and cable tails should be sleeved with insulation suitable for the voltage, ambient and conductor contact temperatures, and colour-coded to indicate polarity, voltage and phase sequence as appropriate.

11.56   In metal trunking housing main cables, special attention should be given to electrical continuity along the route and to earth. Trunking joints should be bonded with tinned copper links of adequate rating, secured across each section.

11.57   Essential services cables should normally be segregated from non-essential services. If segregation is not possible, essential services cables should be fire-resistant and installed with physical barriers.

11.58   Single core three phase conductors in ferrous enclosures should be arranged with the three phases, neutral and earth conductors of the circuit in trefoil or bunched. To prevent the generation of circulating eddy current by single core conductors in the enclosure, the phase conductors must not be separated by internal ferrous barriers or cleats.

Fire-resistant cables

11.59   Mineral insulated cables are available with copper conductors and copper sheaths. Cables having copper conductors and sheaths should comply with BS6207. Armoured and non-armoured cables are also available with copper conductor, silcon rubber or mica-glass tape insulation with extruded xlpe bedding and over-sheath of non-toxic compound. They should comply with BS6724 (armoured) and BS7211 (non-armoured).

11.60   All LV fire-resistant cables must be tested to BS6387 to the class of fire-resistance and temperature required in the installation, as identified by type test and categorised by the following symbols:

a.   resistance to fire only:

(i)   650°C for 3 hours – A;

(ii)   750°C for 3 hours – B;

(iii)   950°C for 3 hours – C;

(iv)   950°C for 20 mins - S;

Optional requirements during period of test:

b.   resistance to fire and water – W;

c.   resistance to fire with mechanical shock:

(i)   650°C – X;

(ii)   750°C – Y;

(iii)   950°C – Z.

11.61   The advantage of mims cables is their proven ability to satisfactorily withstand high or low temperatures and physical impact damage. The powder type mineral insulation used in mims cables readily absorbs moisture up to a maximum of 200 mm into open or badly sealed ends. It is important that the correct seals, fittings and accessories as supplied by the cable manufacturer are used. It is also advisable to use the special installation tools supplied by the cable manufacturer, and to follow their advice concerning need for temporary cable end sealing, during installation.

11.62   The silicon rubber or mica-glass tape-insulated non-toxic cable has the advantage of being easy to handle, flexible for installation, and simpler to terminate. Care must be exercised when handling and terminating to ensure that the outer aluminium screen does not chafe or cut into the soft silicon rubber cable insulation.

Fire alarm circuits

11.63   The main purpose of a fire alarm system is to give an early warning of a fire. Wiring in conduit and trunking is satisfactory for call-points or detectors, as destruction of the call-point or detector connection after initial operation should not affect the sounding of the alarm supplied from the alarm control equipment. The power supply to the alarm control equipment and sounder must be fire-resistant and directly supplied from an essential supply and battery system. BS5839:Part 1 refers.

11.64   General requirements for fire alarm circuits are included in Health Technical Memorandum 82 – 'Firecode: Alarm and detection systems'.

11.65   Circuit wiring, defined by the IEE Wiring Regulations as Category 3, may not be mixed with any other circuits, except in escape lighting wiring.

Polarity of termination

11.66   All terminating cable tails should be numbered or colour-coded to indicate polarity and phase as appropriate.

Cable laying

11.67   Where single core cables are used for heavy current circuits, the cables of the three phases should be laid in close proximity: in trefoil or flat formation, mechanically braced and tied along the route. Care must be taken to reduce eddy currents, for example by the use of non-ferrous clamps, fittings, spacers, gland plates and cable terminations. Single core cables which require armour protection should be armoured with a non-magnetic metal wire or strip and an overall sheath.

11.68   Steel cable trays and aluminium or steel ladder-rack can simplify installation where several cables are to be installed in close proximity. In damp areas and in order to reduce the risk of corrosion by electrolytic or water action, steel trays and ladder-rack should have a protected, galvanised finish.

11.69   HV and LV power and screened control/instrument cables must not be located on the same tray but must be horizontally and/or vertically run on different trays, with a minimum separation of 300 mm. All tray or ladder work should be equibonded and connected to the main earth system.

Cables in conduits

11.70   Cables bunched in steel conduit sizes 20 mm, 25 mm or 32 mm diameter, or in steel trunking will usually represent the most economical type of installation. Conduits smaller than 20 mm diameter should not be used. Trunking has the advantage that it is an adaptable system for subsequent alterations and cable additions. When available, sufficient space should be reserved. Conduit or trunking installations must be completed before cables are pulled.

11.71   The number and sizes of cables pulled into any conduit should not exceed the circuit loading guidance in the IEE Wiring Regulations. The conduit system for each distribution board should be kept separate and cables from different distribution boards should not be enclosed in the same conduit. When it is necessary to pull in cables, the space factor for wiring in ducts should not exceed 35%.

11.72   Conduit should be heavy gauge quality to BS31. Enamel finish is satisfactory for indoor dry locations. A passivated, galvanised, class 4 finish should be specified where damp conditions are likely. Conduit bores must be free of swarf snags and lined with a dry and compatible lubricant. All conduit threads exposed after installation should be coated with a rust-resisting paint. Plastic conduit may only be used in domestic areas or accommodation where electromagnetic interference cannot degrade medical or industrial electrical equipment.

11.73   As far as is practicable, conduits should be continuous between outlets. Factory-made bends, tees, etc should not be used where cable damage would occur due to excessive bending or abrasion while pulling the cables. Conduit fittings should be of malleable cast iron to BS31 or BS4568.

Under-floor steel trunking and duct systems

11.74   Under-floor trunking and duct systems are usually more expensive than alternative methods of installation. There is also a great risk of damage caused by water entering inspection covers of under-floor systems. It is therefore recommended that this system should be used only where there are suitable environmental conditions and safeguards. It is important that the design of equipment floor areas be agreed with the architect and that the structural design provide a concrete floor with an adequate depth of screed to permit any later re-routing or installation of the lay-in ducts or conduit. In certain departments, for example radiotherapy and diagnostic X-ray, it will be necessary to install a level surface over steel conduit or lay-in steel ducts within the floor screed of the main rooms, between the operating panels and the apparatus.

11.75   Where large quantities of data and computer equipment are installed, raised floors with removable square sections to permit sub-floor access for any later cable works are advised.

Steel trunking for cables

11.76   Steel trunking for cables represents the most satisfactory type of installation where a number of circuits can conveniently follow the same path. Cable trunking is suitable for use in voids, above suspended ceilings, surface applications and in vertical ducts. Trunking layouts should be predetermined and be dimensionally co-ordinated with other building components to enable standard prefabricated lengths to be used whenever practicable.

11.77   Complete segregation of non-essential and essential sub-circuit wiring is desirable, but may not be possible in all instances. In the most important areas where the essential installation will include a large number of sub-circuits, it should be a comparatively cheap and simple matter to segregate non-essential circuits from the wiring of essential circuits. In other areas where only a small part of the sub-circuit wiring is connected to the non-essential part of the installation, the additional expense of segregating the essential sub-circuits from non-essential sub-circuits may not be practical or justified.

11.78   A method of achieving this is to use fire-resistant cables throughout, all complying with BS6387.

11.79   Escape lighting circuits for escape routes should always be segregated from both essential and non-essential circuits. Guidance is given in BS5266. Where circuits serving escape lighting in one fire compartment pass through another fire compartment, fire-resistant cable shall be used. Main lighting and domestic power circuits may be installed in the same trunking.

11.80   Extra low voltage circuits can be installed with low voltage circuits operating at mains potential providing that the insulation is equally rated to the maximum circuit voltage present. Wires of mixed service must be suitably screened to reduce inter-circuit electromagnetic interference.

11.81   Small TP and N cables installed in trunking should be tied or clipped together in small convenient bunches. Groups of four single-core larger cables, comprising a 3-phase supply and neutral, should be laid in trefoil, interleaved at suitable intervals and labelled to assist identification of circuits. The number and size of any cable bunch in any trunking should not exceed that allowed in the IEE Wiring Regulations and BS4066 Part 3.

11.82   Cable layout drawings should also include lists of the cables, identified by numbers, which pass through main cable route intersections.

11.83   Metal trunking should have a suitable anti-rust finish (for example zinc-coated sheet or a stove-enamel finish). For damp environments, galvanised trunking should be specified.

11.84   All equipotential contact surfaces must be free of stove enamel or anodised finish to ensure electrical continuity to earth and between trunking sections. Tinned copper bonding links must be used across all trunking section joints to complete the equipotential bond and earth connection. Flexible trunking or conduit must be bridged by a separate equipotential conductor.

11.85   Approved non-flammable fire barriers and penetration seals should be inserted in cable trunking where it penetrates floors and partitions which are themselves intended to form fire barriers. The outside of the trunking should also be locally fire insulated on both sides for 500 mm, to prevent heat transfer by conduction along the metal trunking. Unenclosed cables entering/leaving barriers or seals should also be fire protected with ready mixed inert material or fire-resistant paint.

11.86   Fire barriers and penetration seals must be provided for all cable installations entering/leaving switchrooms, and plant cubicles where gland plate sealing is not provided.

Socket-outlets in sub-circuits

11.87   The prospect of an international plug and socket system has been under discussion by the International Electrotechnical Commission (IEC) since 1967. Progress has been slow towards reaching an accord in design. A system has evolved which has not yet reached the safety standards currently available which comply with BS1363.

11.88   Pending the standardisation of the international socket-outlet, the 13 amp socket-outlets complying with BS1363 for radial or ring main final sub-circuits should be used as a standard throughout HCPs for connecting portable or mobile mains voltage electrical equipment to the supply in medical areas.

11.89   The distribution of socket-outlets in specific departments is dealt with in Hospital Building Notes and the Activity Data Sheets covering those departments, and advice and guidance in HTM 2011 – 'Emergency electrical services'.

11.90   Approved electrical points of supply and equipment are required in those areas where flammable gases or volatile flammable agents are in use. BS5345 refers.

11.91   Generally, the allocation of socket-outlets in corridors should provide for the use of electrically operated cleaning machines assumed to have flexible cords 9 m long. Essential supply and normal supply socket-outlets should be suitably marked as required in HTM 2011 – 'Emergency electrical services'.

11.92   The standardisation of socket-outlets throughout an HCP is considered to be of great importance. There have been instances of delays occurring, with serious consequences, because the plugs on medical-electrical equipment did not match the socket-outlets provided in a particular treatment area. This matter is of special importance when major alterations or extensions are carried out to existing HCPs. Appropriate steps should be taken to standardise all socket-outlets throughout the old and new sections.

Medical-electrical equipment

11.93   This comprises electrical equipment provided with not more than one connection to a mains supply and intended to diagnose, treat or monitor the patient under medical supervision, and which makes physical or electrical contact with the patient and/or transfers energy to or from the patient and/or detects such energy transfer to or from the patient. Medical-electrical equipment and patient safety aspects are dealt with in BS5724:Part 1:1989 – 'Medical electrical equipment' and IEC601-1:1988.

Locations of medical use

An intracardiac procedure is defined as one in which an electrical conductor is placed within the heart of a patient or is likely to come into contact with the heart, such conductor being accessible outside the patient's body. In this context, an electrical conductor includes insulated wires such as cardiac pacing electrodes or intracardiac ECG electrodes, or insulated tubes filled with conducting fluids.

This document, when completed and approved, will be introduced into the IEE Wiring Regulations under part 6 – 'Special installations or locations – particular requirements'.

11.94   These are locations of use where medical equipment is provided with electrical power, directly or indirectly, from the mains supply. An IEC document (IEC 364 – 'Electrical installations of buildings', section 710: "Medical locations") is currently being prepared under the auspices of TC64/WG26 with full participation of the British Electrotechnical Committee. The main proposal of this document will be to classify the HCP into distinct group areas:

a.   Group O: locations where no applied parts of medical-electrical equipment that is supplied from the mains are intended to be used;

b.   Group 1: locations where medical-electrical equipment is intended to be used, but not for intracardiac procedures;

c.   Group 2: locations where medical-electrical equipment for an intracardiac procedure is intended to be used.

Power supply systems in medical areas

11.95   The IEC document refered to in paragraph 11.94 also proposes the following requirements for the supply:

a.   the TN-C system will not be used in medical locations;

b.   TN-S and TT systems may be used in locations 1 or 2 for specific circuits;

c.   an IT system should be used for all mains supplied medical-electrical equipment used for intracardiac procedures. This IT system should comprise an isolating transformer and insulation monitoring devices;

d.   special classification of extra-low voltages to be used in medical locations of Group 2.

LV supplies for high shock risk areas

11.96   A portable 240 V class I (earthed) or, preferably, class II (reinforced insulation, unearthed) appliance which is connected to the mains and used in close proximity to earthed metalwork and/or electrically conducting type floors can constitute a shock risk (for example in service voids, boiler houses and plantrooms). The risk can be reduced by using an RCD, maximum 30 mA setting to BS4293:1983, BS7071 or alternatively a 110 V appliance supplied from a portable step-down class I 240 V/110 V transformer with centre tapped earthed secondary winding to BS3535. The 110 V appliance will require a plug and socket to BS192, that is, with live and return fused at the plug round pins.

11.97   In dry shock risk areas, 240 V/50 V supply transformers with an unearthed secondary winding, complying with BS3535 – 'Safety isolating transformers', should be provided to supply a safety extra low voltage (selv) for use with class III insulated 50 V handlamps or lamp clusters.

11.98   In high shock risk or wet areas, standard mains voltage class II or class I (earthed) hand tools can be fitted with plugs which fit the standard BS1363 socket-outlet, supplied from an inexpensive earth-free supply isolating transformer unit. Figure 11 shows the schematic arrangement of such a unit. Relay A operates at 1 mA, and a person making contact with one of the live lines and earth would pass a maximum current of 3.5 mA, in which event, the supply would be interrupted until the unit were manually reset. A typical rating for such a unit is 500 VA, which would be sufficient for most hand tool applications. The mains input lead to the unit should be kept as short as practicable. This form of protection is advised for 240 V mortuary tools and equipment (see Health Notice HN(82)39).

Cubicle control and indication wiring

11.99   Incoming or outgoing control cable wiring should be suitably insulated, 2.5 mm^2 conductor, comprising seven strands of copper, screened, and preferably operating at a maximum of 110 volts.

11.100   50 V d.c. alarm and indication cable, 1.0 mm diameter conductor twisted pair, coloured and screened, may be routed into and between marshalling boxes, in multi-core cables, to simplify cubicle wiring interconnections.

Service ducts, trenches and tunnels

General

11.101   Duct, trench or tunnel accommodation should make possible the planned site services to be installed with adequate clearances and also include space for possible future requirements.

11.102   As far as is practicable, ducts or trenches for the accommodation of electrical cables should not be used for other services. Where it is necessary to accommodate electrical cables with other services there should be adequate route separation between those services and electric cables or conduits. The electrical cables should be installed in the upper space of a trench or tunnel to minimise the possibility of damage from water. HV cables must not be routed in enclosed areas close to flammable gas or oxygen pipework.

11.103   When sizing ducts, trenches or tunnels, maintenance access should be considered. Small ducts are more difficult for servicing and allow less flexibility as regards alterations and additions. Recommended minimum clearances are given in HTM 23 – 'Access and accommodation for engineering services'.

11.104   Provision of an electrical supply for selv lighting at manholes or access to tunnel entrances and connection of portable ventilation is recommended.

11.105   Where HV cables are installed, they should be identified with "DANGER . . . volts" notices provided at points where access to HV cables can be obtained. Exposed cable installation must always be protected from mechanical damage by barriers, covers or space.

Lift shafts

11.106   Lift shafts should not be used for the accommodation of rising power mains or control systems which are not part of that lift installation.

Construction

11.107 Floors for trenches etc should be constructed of concrete and have a slight fall and a shallow drainage channel with drainage points at suitable intervals. The sides and top covers should be constructed of concrete. Vertical cable ducts or flumes must have fire barriers at each floor level.

11.108 Access openings should be large enough to enable standard lengths of conduit (4.5 m approx) to be installed and removed without bending and should be kept clear of conduits and cables. Figure 17 illustrates the principles that should govern the layout of crawlways, subways and service voids.

External cable runs

11.109 Main cables where directly buried in open ground should be initially laid in, and covered by, sifted soil or sand, and over-covered with reinforced interlocking fibre boards or concrete tiles to BS2484. Boards or tiles afford protection against hand tools but not against mechanical excavators. HV and LV cable routes should be provided with warning tapes, red for HV and yellow for LV cables, and placed 300 mm above the tile or cable. The tapes should not be less than 150 mm wide and 0.1 mm thick and bear the legend "electric cable below" or similar in black letters. They should be made of pvc material which is resistant to the acids or alkalis that may be encountered in the ground. Accurately located concrete surface markers should be provided at intervals of approximately 6.5 m, where practicable, in open ground along the cable route at any change of direction or entry to buildings.

11.110 On main cable routes where additional cables may subsequently be required, spare cable ducts or trench space should be provided. Manholes or access holes should be provided for entry into cable tunnels and ducts. Cable ducts should be used at all points where cables enter buildings. The entry points should be sealed after cable laying to prevent the passage of moisture and vermin.

11.111 Cable ducts should also be used where cables pass under roads or other areas having a permanent made-up surface and should be surrounded with concrete to prevent fracture by traffic. A spare capacity of 25 per cent should be allowed for possible future requirements.

11.112 Cable ducts should be 100 mm minimum diameter bore and made in tough pvc tube or similar approved material, and:

a. each tube should have a plain spigot at one end and a sealing socket in the other end for making a watertight push-fit alignment;

b. the bends of buried ducts may be formed by interconnecting angled socket couplings to obtain the required angle of curvature. A buried duct bend between un-aligned manholes must have a 10 to 15 metre radius of curvature, to minimise cable pull tension;

c. manholes should have drainage and be of adequate dimensions for cable pulling or the installation of traywork, and with tray space for the minimum radius of bending of the largest diameter cable;

d. the loadbearing cable ducts should be immersed in concrete of depth/width to provide a minimum cover of 150 mm above and below and 100 mm on each side of the sockets. The ducts must be secured to prevent flotation in the concrete during pouring;

e. the clearway and alignment of cable ducts should be proved by using a pull-through fitted with an approved test piece (pig) before the enclosing concrete has hardened;

   f. pvc tube must be stored horizontally, shaded from direct sunlight;

   g. recommended minimum buried depths for external cable installations are:

      (i)   low voltage cables – 0.5 m;

      (ii) high voltage cables – 0.8 m.

Cable plan

11.113 A plan print drawing showing accurately the position of all external cable runs, cable ducts and trenches, etc together with all external drainage facilities, should be displayed in a prominent position.

12.0 Switchgear

High voltage switchgear

General

12.1   High voltage circuit breakers for newly designed HCPs will normally be vacuum or SF_6 type, metal-clad, horizontally or vertically isolated, spring or electromagnetically operated, with insulated bus-bars and current transformer chambers in a switchboard enclosure. The current transformers should be the insulated ring type or epoxy resin encapsulated. Switchboards would normally be housed indoors.

12.2   It is important that the symmetrical breaking fault current rating of circuit breakers should exceed the mpfc of the supply system, which should be verified by the regional electricity company (REC).

12.3   An independent NATLAS accredited type test certificate should be obtained from the switchgear manufacturer. Typical rating for an HCP circuit breaker is 250 MVA, 400 amperes at 11 kV.

12.4   For maintenance, provision must be included to earth the three-phase circuit cable terminations through the circuit breaker contacts, preferably from a remote control position. On large HV switchboards, provision should also be made for at least one circuit breaker to earth the bus-bars. Guidance relating to the application of HV safety procedures is given in Health Technical Memorandum 2021 – 'Electrical safety code for high voltage systems ("Operational management")'.

12.5   The Electricity Association provides a standard specification for HV distribution switchgear (EA 41-26: issue 1991) which covers indoor, cable connected metal-clad switchgear ratings up to 36 kV.

12.6   Circuit breakers should be in accordance with British Standards 5486, 5227, 6581, 5311 and 7354, oil switches in accordance with BS5463. The CENELEC EN or IEC standard 947 (many parts) will eventually supersede all BS switchgear documents.

SF_6 and vacuum circuit breakers

12.7   Metal-clad distribution switchgear technology has evolved over many years. Currently, SF_6 (sulphur hexafluoride) and vacuum circuit breakers in the range 11 kV to 33 kV are in common use. The operational and maintenance costs are low, due to the improved methods of arc interruption that both SF_6 contact chambers and vacuum contact interrupters offer.

12.8   The repetitive maintenance required in oil circuit breakers to test and/or change the circuit breaker oil after fault current operation, does not exist in either SF_6 or vacuum types of switchgear. The SF_6 and vacuum circuit breakers contain non-flammable arc interruption media which have given extended fault current-to-break endurance. Fire protection is not required.

12.9 The SF$_6$ circuit breaker three-phase contact chamber is sealed at a pressure of approximately one bar gauge for life, and is maintenance free. In the event of a leak the circuit breaker will still operate safely. In the normal condition of use SF$_6$ is a colourless, odourless, non-toxic, non-flammable gas, with a boiling point of minus 60°C at 760 mm Hg. It is very stable, with excellent heat transfer and dielectric properties during normal contact separation.

12.10 Under catastrophic conditions, in temperatures in excess of 800°C, or when exposed to decomposition by electric arc, free SF$_6$ can produce particulate dust and by-products which can irritate the skin and air breathing passages. These by-products do not all produce the same easily detected and usually strong and nauseous odour.

12.11 Prior to any maintenance work, or following accidents, the equipment and space surrounding must be thoroughly ventilated before any work or inspection is allowed to proceed.

12.12 As a margin of safety, a pressure gauge can be provided, connected to the gas chamber, to monitor gas pressure and to initiate a low pressure alarm and/or set the switching device lockout interlock.

12.13 The SF$_6$ circuit breaker load current arc interruption operation is less aggressive than that of the vacuum circuit breaker, due to the movement of SF$_6$ caused by the mechanism in the opening stroke. The arc interruption extends over one or more cycles and extinguishes at current zero without voltage resonance.

12.14 The vacuum circuit breaker features three separate vaccuum chambers, each with a contact interrupter fitted with its own tripping and wear compensating springs. Contact wear gauges are provided to show when new interrupters are required. The chambers are easily removed after the circuit breaker trolley is withdrawn from the cubicle.

12.15 In vacuum circuit breakers the extinction of the interrupted electric arc is very rapid and can occur several times before the current zero. This causes the phenomenon of "current chopping" which can result in a high transient voltage in an inductive lightly loaded circuit.

12.16 It is recommended that transformers supplied through vacuum circuit breakers be protected by surge arrestors at the circuit breaker cable box terminations.

12.17 In circuit breakers where the SF$_6$ phase chambers or vacuum phase interrupters are separate, a failure in one phase chamber does not prevent the two functioning phase chambers or interrupters breaking the circuit current when the circuit breaker is operated to open.

12.18 Interchangeability between circuit breakers has been developed by some manufacturers to replace oil with vacuum, SF$_6$ with vacuum and vice versa in complete truck units, or air breaker (switching devices) with vacuum or SF$_6$ switching devices. Modifications may be required to the cubicle control wiring and sliding contacts. The extent of interchangeability and availability should be discussed with the manufacturer of the switchboard.

Protection

12.19   It is considered desirable to provide at least idmt overcurrent and instantaneous earth fault protection relays for transformer protection at the main HCP incomer circuit breaker(s). Where compact distribution transformers are connected by ring main unit (RMU) tee-off switching devices, current limiting fuse links or current transformer (CT) operated trip systems should be used.

12.20   For large capacity plant, tapping points should be considered, if available, in either the HV circuit breaker circuit insulation mouldings or cable box terminations. This would assist relay testing by primary injection.

Trip release coil supply

12.21   An earth-free direct current battery charger supply is required to energise the trip coil circuits. An alkaline type battery is normally used for the supply in small installations. In determining the battery voltage, allowance should be made for the voltage drop in the wiring to ensure that the coils operate at their rated voltage. Charging facilities should include an automatic low charging rate, with manually controlled quick charging facilities.

12.22   Manual test facilities or remote trip circuit supervision with alarm should be provided on all HV circuit breakers and relay protected switching devices.

Methods of circuit breaker closure

12.23   Spring closure, the mechanical force required to close and latch a circuit breaker, must be initially greater than the total reaction forces of the rated short-circuit current, and the opening spring. The closure spring is compressed through a mechanical linkage by an a.c. electric motor or a manually operated winding handle. On initiation to close, the potential energy of the closure spring is released.

12.24   Electromagnetic closure, the power energy to close the circuit breaker, is derived from the magnetic force induced by the electrically energised d.c. closing coil. The closing coil armature is connected by mechanical linkages to the circuit breaker closing mechanism. It drives against the opposing forces, which comprise the opening spring, main contact reaction pressures and any short-circuit forces present, if closing onto a fault.

12.25   For mechanical spring closure, a large capacity battery is not required to supply the low power consumption of the trip coils.

12.26   With high power electromagnetic coil closure, the number of repetitive operations to close, multiplied by the number of circuit breakers to be supplied in an emergency, must be considered. Normally a battery within the range 10–25 ampere-hours would be suitable to trip the circuit breaker where closure is spring operated. For repetitive electromagnetic coil closure/opening a larger capacity battery greater than 80 ampere-hours will be necessary. The manufacturer will advise.

12.27   For control voltages of 50 V d.c. and above, resistance or solid positive battery terminal earthing is advised to protect against electrolytic corrosive effects in copper control wires. Battery earth leakage protection should be provided.

12.28   The battery should be housed in a sturdy fire-resisting (for example steel) enclosure. Cables connecting battery and switchgear should have fire-resisting properties and should be segregated from the high voltage and main low voltage feeders. Main fuses should be provided to isolate the battery for maintenance purposes.

12.29   Separate isolating trip links and closure fuses should be provided at each circuit breaker.

Current transformers

12.30   Current transformers (CTs) for use with protective and measuring equipment should comply with BS3938.

12.31   The CT winding ratio and secondary magnetisation output currents chosen should extend over the full load current operating and instrument ranges. The primary winding current ratio should be equal to, or the first standard ratio above, the load current. Two ratios may be incorporated in one CT design, to adapt to later system planned uprating.

12.32   The linear portion of the magnetisation curve should be used. The point of saturation (knee point) must exceed the following different operating requirements:

a.   full load current metering;

b.   or alternatively, the more costly CT for maximum fault current levels required in protection over-current relays and instantaneous hi-set trip settings.

12.33   The secondary current ratings are normally 1 ampere or 5 amperes at full load.

12.34   The specific accuracy of instrument CTs is given as a percentage of the primary current ratio, coded in classes as:

a.   (.1) = 0.15% [AL];

b.   (.2) = 1.0% [AM];

c.   (0.5) = 1.0–1.5% [BM];

d.   (1.0) = 1.0–2.5% [CM];

e   (3.0) = 10.0% [C].

The square bracketed letters [ ] above indicate the earlier accuracy codes

This covers the ranges of most scientific, precision and commercial requirements.

12.35   Accuracy of protection CTs are classified as:

a.   (5P) = 1.0% [S];

b.   (10P) = 3.0% [T].

12.36   The burden of the CT is largely determined by the type of load expressed in VA. Ammeters are typically 2 VA, while more complex instruments can be up to 10 VA. The secondary current rating can be either 1 ampere or 5 amperes. For long wire runs the 1 ampere CT is more suitable. The wire burden varies with the current (squared) for an equal wire conductor.

12.37   The 1 ampere secondary winding current transformer will also permit the use of a 10 ampere a.c. multimeter for secondary injection protection tests.

Voltage transformers

12.38   The voltage transformers (VTs) for use with protective and measuring equipment should comply with BS3941.

12.39   The VT may be star-star connected for instruments or star-open delta for protection circuits. It is used in HV systems operating up to 66 kV, and provides a secondary output to relays and measuring equipment at a standardised (UK) low voltage of 63.5 V per phase (110 V line).

12.40   Accuracy should be selected to suit instrumentation or protection requirements. Load ratings are typically small (200 VA). The step-down ratios are large, and hence the primary currents correspondingly small at a few milliamperes.

12.41   With such small currents it is not practical to provide a fine wire HV fuse link to protect for all possible faults. A balanced compromise is recommended between a wire to suit the primary fault current and, alternatively, a possible wire metal fatigue. This is to give better reliability of supply at the equipment, with a fuse link value between 2-3 amperes at all the HV levels. Low voltage fuse links are also included to provide protection to the equipment and LV instrument connections.

Interlocks, safety shutters and labelling

12.42   Mechanical interlocks, safety shutter devices, unique locks and keys, earthing equipment and labelling should be provided and approved as specified in HTM 2021 – 'Electrical safety code for high voltage systems' and in statutory requirements.

High voltage SF$_6$ ring main units

12.43   SF$_6$ switches are considerably cheaper to maintain than oil immersed fuse switches. The two fault making switches and tee-off switch are enclosed and sealed for life in cast epoxy-resin modules containing the SF$_6$ atmosphere. They may be equipped with protection of hrc current limiting fuse links or current transformer operated trip coils to suit the tee-off transformer rating. The SF$_6$ pressure is set to suit the rating, approx 0.35 bar gauge.

High voltage ring main oil immersed fused switches

12.44   Oil fused switches are about two-thirds of the cost of a comparable circuit breaker. They require routine examination and change of the oil with use and age. They are normally equipped with hrc current limiting fuses complying with BS2692 and are suitable for protection where time discrimination is required.

Heaters

12.45   Low-rated wire-wound resistance heaters should be located in each HV circuit breaker or switching device cubicle, where switchrooms are subjected to weather exposure, ambient swings in temperature, or in areas of high relative humidity. Switchroom space heating may be inadequate.

Low voltage switchboards

General

12.46   Switchboards and panels should be designed with surrounding space to give flexibility for access and end extension. Separation of internal parts should be specified in the required forms 1, 2, 3 and 4 detailed in BS5486.

12.47 The bus-bars, switches and fuse-gear should be rated for the mpfc of the system. Where the supply is obtained direct from the REC's high voltage sub-station or low voltage network, the mpfc should be verified with the REC and the rating specified accordingly.

12.48 Experience has shown that air break switches complying with BS EN 60947-3:1992 and air break LV circuit breakers complying with BS4752 have been generally satisfactory.

12.49 IEC 947 will replace the existing BS and IEC specifications and be adopted as the European Norm (EN) document (see "References").

12.50 IEC 947 will introduce important changes in low voltage switchgear design, such as:

- new utilisation categories;
- revised ratings with new definitions;
- revision of short circuit ratings;
- changes in overload current capacities;
- re-allocation of rated currents;
- new definition for protection discrimination.

12.51 MCB, MCCB and contactor type switch devices are defined as "open type", where the interrupting medium is air. When specifying a circuit breaker the exact requirement must be more precise.

12.52 An isolation device is redefined as a disconnector (that is, without load breaking capacity) or as a switch disconnector (that is, with load breaking capacity), and a fuse-switch as a fuse combination switch.

Fuse-switches and isolators

12.53 Fuse-switches and isolators are normally three-phase, with moving double break contacts and a fixed neutral link. The neutral may be provided also as a moving contact if specified.

12.54 The current ratings range from 63 to 800 amperes and they are fault rated to 50 kA. The fuse-switch has three-phase fuse links provided. They are located between the double break contacts and move with the operation of the open-close mechanism. The open-close mechanism may be integral with the cubicle door, and the moving contacts and fuse links may be exposed for inspection when the cubicle door is unbolted and hinged outwards from the shrouded, fixed contacts after the mechanism is operated to open.

12.55 The isolator does not have fuse links attached to the moving mechanism, but it may be a modified fuse-switch with solid links replacing the fuse links to give a double break isolation. Isolators are available also with single break. A locking facility must be provided for securing the isolator or fuse-switch in the open position.

12.56 Fuse-switches and isolators can be provided in tiered cubicles, the number limited by the fixed height of the cubicle and the physical dimensions of the switch. The incomer to the cubicle may be an air circuit breaker or fuse-switch.

Motor starters

12.57   When conforming to IEE Wiring Regulations, protection co-ordination is provided by upstream hrc current limiting fuses and a motor overload thermal relay. The motor relay generally provides protection to both the motor and the cable, as the cable will be sized to the motor rating. The fuse will provide short circuit protection to the cable and the starter assembly. BS EN 60947-4-1:1992 – 'Motor starters' describes three types of starter protective co-ordination, as follows:

a.   type a – damage to contactor and overload relay permitted, provided enclosure remains intact and provides complete protection to individuals;

b.   type b – permits overload trip to be altered permanently without other damage or injury to individuals;

c.   type c – does not permit damage to overload relay or contactor or injury to individuals.

12.58   Light welding of type b and c contacts is acceptable if the welds can be easily broken. It is apparent that type c is the preferred design.

12.59   In IE 947-4, types a, b and c are replaced by types 1 and 2. Type 1 corresponds to type a, and type 2 corresponds almost to type c as the requirement is applicable to the overload relay, that is, the contactor can fail providing the contacts are separable or replaceable. Type 2 test should include major short-circuit tests, make and break test and overload calibration test. The fault rating of starters will change from the present 1 second duration to a range of times in multiples of 50 milliseconds.

12.60   Where possible, direct comparison should be sought with the new certified ratings. Existing starters will require re-certification.

12.61   For safe live control and alarm circuit tests, motor starter isolators should incorporate a "Test" position. The 415 V three-phase supply to the starter and motor terminals is then isolated, but maintains the control and alarm voltage supplies.

Motor protection

12.62   Motor protection should be arranged to provide adequate discrimination between the supply cable and motor winding (see paragraph 20.7).

12.63   Where electric motors or generators provide an essential service or supply for ventilation, refrigeration, lifts, and fire equipment to the HCP, a continuously operating device to measure the insulating resistance of the three-phase winding is advised. This device should have winding low insulating resistance alarm and control lockout facility.

Reduced voltage starting

12.64   The most common conventional method of reduced voltage starting of a.c. induction motors is the star-delta method. This is a two-step method which initially connects the motor winding terminals in star, then changes over to the motor final connection of delta after a pre-determined rotational accelerating time has elapsed. The voltage across each winding is in star, which is the phase voltage (V_p). This initial lower voltage reduces the start current surge that would result from a direct on-line voltage (V_l) as at a delta connected motor winding, but the time to accelerate will be increased. The starting torque of an induction motor is proportional to the square of the winding voltage. For a star, three-phase connected winding, the starting torque is reduced to V_p^2/V_l^2, that is, to one-third of the starting torque in a delta winding at normal voltage V_1. All six winding ends are separately terminated at the motor terminal bar, and from there, by six cable cores to the starter cable box.

12.65   Star-delta starters require three sets of three-phase contactors:

a.   main contactor;

b.   to connect winding in star;

c.   to connect winding in delta;

d.   a timer to initiate changeover from star to delta connection at a suitable point on the speed/torque characteristic.

12.66   Alternatively, where a low starting current and gradually increasing starting (or stopping) torques are required, a method of starting can be used which requires a thyristor, controller and a basic on-line starter, connected to an induction motor in delta. The input voltage can be ramp increased over a pre-selected time interval of up to 60 seconds maximum, depending upon the thyristor thermal capacity.

12.67   The induction motor can be controlled to give a smooth accelerating speed against the load torque, as the winding voltage is increased.

12.68   The motor can also be run at sub-synchronous speeds by variation of the thyristor controlled ramp voltage, with the following advantages:

a.   for a required revs/min and load torque, the thyristor adjusts the stator input voltage. This changes the magnetising current, the main inductive reactive current component, in magnitude relative to the active current component which provides the load torque requirement. This combined effect maximises the induction motor low load power factor, and minimises motor iron and copper losses;

b.   reduced voltage starting may be ineffective with high torque loads, for example compressors. Expert advice should be sought.

Heaters

12.69   Low rated wirewound heaters may be required in highly rated LV circuit breakers, contactor cubicles, or motor control centres where ambient conditions are variable.

Cable glands and terminations

12.70   The choice of a suitable cable gland and termination is all-important in bonding the cable and the equipment into a reliable, long-lasting connection and weatherproof seal. Glands should be made to BS6121 and terminations to BS4579 and BS EN 609-47-1:1992.

12.71   The choice and size of gland must be in accord with the environmental conditions, the cable box, gland plate, type of cable to be terminated and the method of earthing to be applied between the cable and equipment. Cable and armour should be secured by a locking ring for a double earth bond if a tapped gland plate entry is not used.

12.72   Special care must be taken in securing gland nuts that may be loosened by shock loading, for example X-ray equipment, subject to current impulse.

12.73   The overall cable diameter and material used will be influenced by the applied voltage, current, physical and environmental conditions of the cable route, as follows:

a.   large current flows will mean that more than one cable may be required for each phase in a circuit. Even so, several smaller cables at a gland-plate entry should each be prospective fault current rated equal to or greater than that of the equipment;

b.   the cable outer diameter must be within the gland manufacturer's recommended tolerance for a particular type and size of gland. This ensures the required weather protection to BS EN 60947-1:1992 and BS EN 60529:1992;

c.   the gland-plate size and cable box will be influenced by the size and type of cable, the total number of circuit cable entries, and the minimum clearance to earth and between phases;

d.   tool access to the inner and outer gland securing nuts must be possible after the cables are passed through the gland and gland-plate.

12.74   A list of cable glands available is shown in Table 5. Table 6 shows the gland/cable designation key.

LV gland selection guide (BS6121)

Cable type		Unarmoured		Metal armoured/braided, including strip aluminium, AWA, copper or steel braided					OCMA type PVC, LC, SWA, TYL
		A1/A2	Nylon	B	C	D1	Barrier	E1	
Operating conditions		Outer seal	Outer seal	No seal	Outer seal	Inner seal	Inner barrier and outer seal	Inner and outer seals	Inner and outer seals
Indoor	Clear and dry	X	X	X	X	X	X	X	X
	Humid	X	X	O	X	I	X	X	X
	Dusty	X	I	I	X	X	X	X	X
Outdoor	Oily	X	X	I	I	X	X	X	X
	Protected	X	X	O	X	I	X	X	X
	Exposed	X	O	O	X	I	X	X	X

Table 5   X – gland suitable; O – gland not suitable; I – gland suitable when correctly fitted.

Cable type	SWA	Aluminium strip armour	Wire braided	Unarmoured and OCMA
Gland designation suffix	W	Y	X	
Flameproof gland suffix	WF	YF	X	F

Table 6 Gland/cable designation key.

12.75 Standard cable glands are manufactured to BS6121 and mineral insulated cable glands to BS6081. Gland materials are:

a. standard brass to BS2874;

b. aluminium to BS1474;

c. wrought steel to BS970.

12.76 The preferred gland threads are ISO (metric) to BS3643. Adaptors for thread incompatibility or to form integral insulated barriers are available from manufacturers. Glands with integral earth or loose earth tags are available. Weather protection, pvc gland shrouds and nickel plating should be used on all gland installations in hostile environments.

12.77 Earth bonding for LV is normally achieved at the gland to the gland-plate screwed entry, and/or at the cable by the gland nut compression locking ring or cone onto the cable armour. In HV and in some instances LV this may not be considered adequate, and integral earth lugs or earth tags should be incorporated into the gland assembly and bonded to the equipment mainframe earth.

12.78 Large LV motors (100 amp-plus ratings), all generators and HV equipment must be frame earthed by adequately rated protective conductors connected directly into the main earth system.

12.79 Cable glands with integral insulated barriers are required where single core cable armour or screen induced circulating currents will derate the cable or cause false current levels in protection current transformers. In such cases the integral insulated part of the gland can be fitted as a loose adaptor item at the time of cable glanding.

12.80 Cable box terminations are usually of the lug and stud type or the ferrule and clamp type. It is essential that lugs or ferrules are the correct fit, to suit cable conductor diameter and stranding, and to prevent loose fitting or overstressed compression in the metal-to-metal bonding surface.

12.81 Outdoor cable box terminations of LV power cables should be sealed with anti-corrosion and anti-tracking protection, by:

a. encapsulation;

b. plastic, heat-shrinkable sleeve;

c. approved grease; or

d. lacquer covering.

12.82 All terminations should be clearly marked for later identification to BS5559.

Bus-bars and chambers

12.83   Bolted or clamped joints can be made on copper bus-bars. The following requirements should be met for obtaining a good joint:

a.   the surface of the metal must be clean and free of oxide;

b.   air and moisture must be excluded from the joint to prevent reformation of oxide, preferably by tinning. Tinning the contact surface of the copper work at the manufacturing stage is a more controlled method than the application of jointing compound at site assembly;

c.   a uniform contact pressure must be applied and maintained;

d.   the bolts should be torque spanner-tightened. The pressure of contact is important. The degree of bolt tension and hence compression of the bus-bar may be influenced also by the material used in the bolt washers. As a general guide, a desirable minimum pressure is 5.5 MN/m^2 (800 lb/in^2).

12.84   Bus-bar enclosures should only contain wiring which connects directly to the associated current transformers. Bus-bars and bus-bar connections should comply with BS159 and BS5486.

Meters and instruments

12.85   The supply to the main distribution switchboard should be equipped with an ammeter and four suitably rated current transformers, one in each phase and neutral, together with a selector switch to enable the current loading of each phase, and the neutral, to be selected using one ammeter, and:

a.   ammeters should be located in all major circuits. A voltmeter should also be specified together with a selector switch to allow the voltages between each phase and to neutral to be selected;

b.   kilowatt-hour meters should be suitable for unbalanced loads, be capable of producing pulsed outputs for centralised reading, and comply with BS5685. The use of kilowatt-hour meters for individual departmental costing must be justified;

c.   indicating instruments should comply with BS89 industrial grade. 100 mm dial instruments are normally considered satisfactory;

d.   current transformers for use with instruments should comply with BS3938;

e.   voltage transformers, if provided, should comply with BS3941.

12.86   All instrument full-scale-indicated deflections should compare with rated secondary current ratios of the connected current transformer or voltage transformer.

Sub-distribution centres

12.87   Sub-distribution switchgear and distribution boards should be situated so as to minimise the length of circuit wiring. Switch and fusegear space enclosures should be well ventilated and accessible. The enclosure and area must not be used for any non-electrical purpose and should have adequate fire-resisting separation at wall, floor and ceiling levels and with any corridor or staircase forming a recognised means-of-escape route. Distribution switchboards should, where practicable, be situated to enable working access from a standing and arm's-length position. Switchable lighting should be provided to enable fuse board work at all times of the day, and be designed to illuminate the vertical surfaces.

12.88   All individual switches, fuse-switches and fuse boards should be clearly and indelibly labelled to indicate the circuits controlled or parts of the healthcare premises supplied. As far as is practicable a standard form of laminated plastic labelling should be used throughout the installation.

12.89   Distribution and sub-distribution enclosure doors should be fitted with entry locks to prevent unauthorised interference, the locks being of common combination throughout the installation. Where distribution equipment is not in a locked enclosure or switchroom, a lock should be fitted to each distribution board. A provision to lock the supply switch **open**, to isolate every distribution sub-distribution fuse board, is required for safety at work.

12.90   Spare ways (for example 25%) and fuses should be provided and space allowed for future additional unequipped units in all fuse/MCB distribution panels.

Feeder pillars

12.91   In new healthcare premises, it will be possible to make indoor facilities available to house sub-distribution equipment. Instances may arise where it will be convenient and economical to employ outdoor feeder pillars, where a feeder is used to supply several peripheral buildings, for example staff accommodation or workshops.

12.92   Details of cable terminations, bus-bars and all statutory safety arrangements (including the shielding of bus-bars and live connections and, where necessary, anti-condensation heating) should be covered by specification.

13.0 High voltage sub-stations

Siting

13.1   Although it is desirable to site sub-stations as near as possible to the load centre to be served, it is also necessary to consider the fire risk to other parts of the healthcare premises and nuisance of noise from circuit breakers, alarms and transformers, particularly during the night hours. Whenever practicable, sub-stations should not be located in main premises or buildings and always be far enough away from wards and operating theatre suites to avoid any possibility of noise nuisance.

13.2   Where practicable, transformer sub-stations should be installed protected from the weather, at ground level. Mineral oil-cooled transformers should only be installed at ground level.

13.3   Because of restricted access for fire-fighting and the possibility of flooding, basement sites should be avoided.

13.4   Air-cooled dry type transformers have more flexibility with regard to location in buildings, as the windings are fire-retardant. Mineral oil-cooled transformers should **not** be located below or next to normally habitable areas in building complexes.

Access and exit

13.5   Sub-stations should be accessible from a road to allow easy access for transformer changing, fire appliances, maintenance vehicles, etc. There are safety restrictions for personnel access to high voltage sub-stations and the provision of emergency exit doors of the approved "crash bar" type. These must be provided at regular 20 m intervals, and located in suitable places to prevent entrapment of personnel.

Layout

13.6   The cable trench layout should allow adequate space for pulling in and terminating cables, and wall clearances for servicing switchgear or cubicles. The size of the sub-station should be related to the anticipated total development, either by allowing unequipped extension for future additions or by locating and designing the sub-station so that future building extension is possible.

13.7   Headroom should be sufficient to ensure adequate natural cooling and space for luminaires and fire protection equipment. Typical layouts are shown in Figures 14-17. A work space should be provided at the end of the switchboard for maintenance work on at least one circuit breaker. It is not necessary to provide sufficient headroom and a lifting beam to facilitate the removal of a transformer from its tank while inside the chamber. In the event of an equipment fault it must be possible for the transformer to be moved into the open air and a crane used.

13.8   Ring anchor fixing should be available for hauling transformers into position or out to the open air.

13.9   The cable entries and ducts should be routed to avoid obstruction in the removal of the transformer.

13.10   The following minimum clearances are recommended:

   a.   between transformer and wall – 1.0 m;

   b.   headroom above transformer tank – 1.6 m;

   c.   headroom above switchboard – 0.9 m;

   d.   between rear of HV and LV switchgear and wall – 0.8 m;

   e.   at front of LV switchboard – 1 m vertically, and to the wall 2 m, for horizontally isolated switching devices.

13.11   As far as is practicable all equipment instruments and protection relays should be accessible from floor level. Operational equipment beyond normal height or reach should be provided with a suitable access platform.

Construction

13.12   The minimum construction requirements are:

   a.   walls and fire-resisting partitions forming the chamber must comply with statutory Building Regulations or equivalent fire-resisting steel fabricated modular construction. Internal walls should have a suitable finish to reduce dust formation and facilitate cleaning;

   b.   floors and ceilings must be reinforced concrete or equivalent fire-resisting construction. Floors should have a non-slip, dust reducing finish;

   c.   doors should open outwards and the width of the opening should allow sufficient clearance for transformers;

   d.   to minimise solar heat gain, windows should not be provided in transformer chambers.

Oil/fluid retaining arrangements for transformers

13.13   Transformer chambers which will house synthetic fluid or mineral oil-cooled transformers should have retaining walls or similar provision, and be finished to prevent fluid/oil spreading in the event of leakage. Retaining arrangements should be capable of holding more than the total fluid/oil content of the transformers and are preferable to underground sumps. The cable and retaining arrangements should not impede the removal of the transformer.

Ducts

13.14   Cable trenches and ducts should be constructed to avoid paths along which surface water, leaking mineral oil or synthetic fluid will flow. All indoor/outdoor connecting cable trenches into which a leakage path is likely, that is, cable entries and exits at and below ground level, should have the edges around the outside covers sealed with a suitable weather sealant. All outside cable trench covers should be sealed against water penetration.

13.15   Cable trenches and ducts should have a fire-resisting barrier (for example expanded fire-resisting foam, gravel or sand blocks) where they pass beneath walls and through partitions which themselves form fire-resisting barriers in or between parts of the building.

13.16 External cable ducts, where they enter buildings, should be sealed to prevent ingress of water and entry of vermin.

Fire protection

Fire-resisting separation and extinguishing equipment is not required for vacuum or SF$_6$ circuit breakers, nor dry type nor Formel NF fluid-filled transformers.

13.17 The fire risk associated with existing mineral oil circuit breakers and transformers is slight, but it is important that reasonable precautions are taken to contain an oil leak or electrical explosion and to prevent the spread of a fire. In addition to the fire-resisting separation between transformer chambers and switchrooms, there should be open ground separation between these areas and healthcare areas of the premises. Where this cannot be arranged, fixed automatic fire extinguishing apparatus and fire-resisting blastwall protection should be provided. Fixed fire-extinguishing equipment need not be provided where each transformer or switchboard is housed in a sub-station or building not part of the main building or premises.

13.18 High voltage and low voltage cables should be installed in separate ducts or conduits, or at different tray levels with 300 mm separation between them. A segregated route should be provided for low voltage feeders, essential or emergency supply cables near where transformers are installed.

13.19 Tripping and closing control circuit cables which are external to circuit breakers should be resistant to fire damage. Fire barriers should be provided where cables pass through fire-resistant partitions or walls.

Fire-extinguishing apparatus

13.20 Where required, transformer chambers should have an automatic fire-extinguishing system when housing mineral oil-cooled transformers. HV switchrooms containing oil circuit breakers, with or without fire barrier protection between bus-bars and switchboards, should be equipped with a CO$_2$ fire-extinguishing installation arranged with overhead fusible links, set to operate at 68°C. The CO$_2$ link line connecting to the dead weight should consist of non-ferrous flexible cord installed in 20 mm diameter galvanised steel conduit. On operating at temperature, the link lines connected to the dead weight device are severed at a fusible link. The fall of the dead weight opens the CO$_2$ cylinder isolating seals in a non-reversible operation, which empties all the CO$_2$ cylinders.

13.21 The CO$_2$ operating mechanism must have a manual locking pin arrangement to prevent the dead weight falling when switchroom access by personnel is required. No person may enter a switchroom when the CO$_2$ is in an operative state.

13.22 Indicating green/red lamps and a remote alarm should be provided to indicate when the CO$_2$ mechanism is inoperative or operative. The entrances to all switchrooms with CO$_2$ fire-extinguishing equipment should be clearly marked with the appropriate warning signs. A manual release should also be provided which should be housed in a glass-fronted box mounted outside the access door to the chamber. It should be painted red and its use clearly indicated.

13.23 If Halon gas fire-extinguishing equipment has been installed instead of CO$_2$, then the same precautionary safety requirements are necessary. Halon is a chlorofluorocarbon type gas and must be phased out from further use by the year 2000.

13.24   The cylinders of liquified CO_2 or Halon should comply with BS5045 and should be mounted vertically in a suitable rack located outside the fire risk area. The quantity of CO_2 should be on the basis of one 45 kg cylinder for each 45 m^3 of room volume to be protected. Discharge nozzles should be located at a high level and connected to the release valve by means of steel piping complying with BS1387, galvanised heavy quality type. The spacing of discharge nozzles will depend on the type selected, and should be arranged in accordance with the manufacturer's recommendations.

Ventilation

13.25   Transformer chambers should be adequately ventilated direct to the outer air to prevent excessive temperature rise. Transformer losses are indicated in Table 7.

Rating kVA	Transformer type	Relative cost	No load loss (W)	Load loss (W at 75°C)	Total mass (Kg)	Im-pedance volts (%)	Mean level sound dB (A)*
315	Oil-filled	100	700	4800	1524	4.75	50
	Midal-filled	+125	700	4800	1524	4.75	50
	Silicon-filled	+120	700	4800	1524	4.75	50
	Formel-filled	+115	700	4800	1540	4.75	—
	Air-cooled "C"	+200	1250	4935	1640	5.00	—
500	Oil-filled	100	1030	6860	2270	4.75	52
	Midal-filled	+125	1030	6860	2270	4.75	52
	Silicon-filled	+120	1030	6860	2270	4.75	52
	Formel-filled	+115	1030	6860	2090	4.75	—
	Air-cooled "C"	+200	1600	5640	2200	5.00	—
	Cast resin	+200	1340	5700	2350	4.00	62
800	Oil-filled	100	1500	10000	3200	4.75	54
	Midal-filled	+125	1500	10000	3200	4.75	54
	Silicon-filled	+120	1500	10000	3200	4.75	54
	Formel-filled	+115	1500	10000	2900	4.75	—
	Air-cooled "C"	+200	2300	7980	2420	5.00	—
	Cast-resin	+200	1700	8300	3000	6.00	63
1000	Oil-filled	100	1770	11800	3850	4.75	55
	Midal-filled	+125	1770	11800	3850	4.75	55
	Silicon-filled	+120	1770	11800	3850	4.75	55
	Formel-filled	+115	1770	10800	3200	4.75	—
	Air-cooled "C"	+200	2350	8400	3310	5.00	—
	Cast resin	+200	2250	8400	3900	6.00	63

* BS6056:1991

Table 7   Comparison of transformers with copper windings (11 kV) (figures are approximate)

13.26   Where practicable, the ventilation should be arranged with low-level inlet openings on one side of the chamber, and high-level openings on the other side or in the roof to ensure good cross-ventilation over the transformer cooling tubes.

13.27   As a general guide, a ratio of 0.1 m^2 of inlet and outlet ventilation openings to each 100 kVA of transformer capacity is suggested. It is frequently convenient to provide louvres in the lower part of external doors for the input ventilation, with high-level wall mounted louvres or penthouse louvres as outlet ventilation.

13.28 High voltage switchrooms should also have permanent inlet and outlet ventilation direct to the outer air. Extract fans should be installed, where considered necessary, to regulate ambient temperature and maintain a low level of humidity.

13.29 In switchrooms with CO_2 (or Halon) fire protection, inlet and outlet ventilating air dampers should be provided to close by spring release, initiated by the separation of fusible links set to melt at an ambient temperture of 68°C.

Heating

13.30 To reduce the possibility of condensation, HV switchrooms should be provided with thermostatically controlled heating which is capable of maintaining the temperature of the switchroom at not less than 10°C with an outdoor temperature of 0°C. Where electric heating is used, the heaters should be permanently installed and should be of a totally enclosed low temperature type.

Lighting

13.31 Adequate levels of illumination should be provided in the equipment rooms. The suggested average level of illumination in the high voltage switchroom and transformer chamber is 150 lux at floor level. The luminaires in the switchroom should be arranged to give good illumination to the front, rear and vertical surfaces of the switchboard. Multiway switching should be provided at all door access points to the switchroom. Emergency escape and standby non-maintained lighting must be provided.

Socket-outlets

13.32 An adequate number of standard 13 amp mains socket-outlets should be provided at the front and rear of switchboards. Portable safe extra low voltage transformers should be used to supply handlamps.

Telephones

13.33 A telephone with facilities for communication through the healthcare premises telephone switchboard should be provided in each HV sub-station.

Warning notices

13.34 Conspicuous and indelible notices reading "DANGER – high voltage" should be provided on lockable doors to rooms containing, or on lockable doors giving access to, high voltage equipment. Sub-stations should be identified with a number or letter.

13.35 A safety notice reading "CO_2" (or "Halon") in red letters on a white background should be fixed on the outside of lockable doors giving access to rooms having CO_2 or Halon installations in addition to the safety signs, prohibition and warning notices complying with BS5378.

13.36 An extract from the management HV safety rules and a safety poster with first-aid treatment for persons suffering from electric shock should be exhibited in each sub-station. Refer to Health Technical Memorandum 2021 – 'Electrical safety code for high voltage systems'.

Mimic diagram and key locker

13.37 A mimic diagram and key locker should be provided at the main high voltage sub-station/switchroom designated for the system. HTM 2021 refers.

Elimination of piped services

13.38 The routing of any pipes through, above or into switchrooms should be avoided, except in the case of a CO_2 or Halon installation.

14.0 Low voltage switchrooms

Siting

14.1   Switchrooms other than those associated with sub-stations should be sited as close as possible to the load centre and arranged to allow convenient direct entry to rising ducts, horizontal ducts, crawlways, etc.

Layout

14.2   The layout should allow adequate space around the switchboard for servicing purposes. Suggested minimum clearances between the switchboard and walls are 0.8 m minimum at the rear and 1 m in front, plus additional space recommended by the manufacturer for withdrawing switchgear. Where provision is made for bus-bars to be extended, adequate space should be allowed at one end of the switchboard for this purpose.

14.3   A single-line diagram should be painted across the switchboard panels, with the relevant plant symbols in voltage-representative colours, for easy guidance in the bus-bar/connecting plant arrangement.

Floor

14.4   The floors should have a non-slip, dust reducing finish.

Walls

14.5   As a minimum requirement, internal walls should be fair-faced brickwork, painted to reduce dust formation and facilitate cleaning. Highly flammable wall finishes should be avoided. Walls and doors should be constructed to fire regulations and standard statutory requirements.

Trenches

14.6   Under-floor trenches with removeable covers will normally be required to accommodate incoming and distribution cables. Fire barrier protection must be provided in outgoing trenches, ducts and main equipment within the switchroom.

14.7   Outdoor cable trench covers should be sealed down with hot, poured bitumen where there is a danger of water penetration into the switchroom.

Separation of supplies

14.8   Where the switchboard consists of two or more main sections with interconnection switchgear for emergency use only, the main feeder cables should be kept as far apart as is practicable to reduce the possibility of a fault on one service affecting the other service cables.

Rubber mats

14.9   Rubber mats complying with BS921 should be provided along the front of the switchboard.

Heating

14.10   To reduce the possibility of condensation, low voltage switchrooms should be provided with thermostatically controlled heating designed to prevent the temperature falling below 10°C with an outdoor temperature of 10°C. Where electric heating is used the heaters should be of totally enclosed low temperature type.

Ventilation

14.11   The switchroom should be provided with permanent inlet and outlet ventilation direct to the outer air.

Lighting

14.12   A good standard of illumination should be provided in the low voltage switchroom. A minimum of 150 lux at floor level in the working area is suggested. The luminaires should be arranged to give good illumination of the front, rear and vertical surfaces of the switchboards. Multiway switching should be provided at all door access points to the switchroom.

14.13   Emergency escape and standby lighting must be provided.

Socket-outlets

14.14   An adequate number of standard 13 amp mains socket-outlets should be provided at the front and rear of switchboards. Portable safe extra low voltage transformers should be used to connect handlamps.

Telephones

14.15   A telephone with facilities for communication through the HCP telephone switchboard should be provided in each switchroom.

Marking

14.16   All switching devices should be clearly and indelibly marked by screwed-on engraved labels indicating the circuits controlled. Labels marked "DANGER 415 VOLTS" etc should be provided on panels etc enclosing live conductors operating at LV potentials.

Wiring diagram

14.17   A schematic single-line diagram, black on white framed and glazed, should be provided at a conspicuous position in the switchroom to show clearly the function of all switches and fuse-gear. This will assist in clearing faults with the minimum of delay.

Spares and tools

14.18   Adequate spare fuses and other essential spare parts, rubber gloves complying with BS697, and any circuit breaker special tools which are liable to be required for emergency use should be provided in a special cabinet or other reserved place.

Safety poster

14.19   A safety poster with first-aid treatment for persons suffering from electric shock should be exhibited in each 415 V switchroom. Refer to HTM 2020 – 'Electrical safety code for low voltage systems'.

Elimination of piped services

14.20   The routing of any pipes through or into the switchrooms should be avoided.

15.0 Transformers

High voltage transformers

Types of transformer

15.1   Four methods of cooling transformer windings are available, namely:

a   mineral insulating oil-cooled, free breathing or sealed;

b.   synthetic insulating fluid-cooled (Formel NF, Midal and Silicon), free breathing or sealed;

c.   dry open air-cooled;

d.   dry cast resin air-cooled.

15.2   Synthetic insulating fluid-cooled transformers cost approximately 40% more than mineral oil-cooled. The dry open type costs approximately 80–100% more than mineral oil-cooled. The dry cast resin type costs approximately 80% more than mineral oil-cooled. Manufacturers should be consulted for the latest price variations. Other typical comparisons of these transformers are given in Table 7.

Fire assessment

15.3   In considering the overall economics of the four types it is necessary to take into account the fire risks and the related environmental hazards. Fire precaution measures can be a significant cost factor with transformers which are installed in indoor sub-stations. Environmental hazards to all personnel must be considered in the event of fire, and logistical contingency measures should be ready in the event of a spillage inside the enclosure area.

15.4   The construction and layout of a sub-station suitable for mineral oil and synthetic fluid cooled sealed tank transformers, and the appropriate fire precautions, are dealt with in paragraph 13.17.

15.5   Oil-cooled transformers have been extensively used and experience has shown them to be very reliable. The only real disadvantage is the high flammability of the mineral insulating oil. Oil-cooled transformers should only be installed at ground floor level. They should never be located below habitable areas, and should have an automatic fire-extinguishing system when housed near habitable or enclosed locations.

15.6   In high fire risk areas within the main premises, both the dry open air-cooled and cast resin air-cooled type transformers are suitable. The Formel NF synthetic fluid-cooled transformer provides a choice for high fire risk areas in outdoor locations. In intermediate fire risk areas, the Midal silicon synthetic fluid-cooled transformers provide a second alternative choice.

Number of transformers

15.7   The number of main supply transformers required for an HCP power system will depend on the load and the extent of the distribution network. A minimum of two transformers should be considered, with a system of cross-connected emergency switching included to enable a supply to be maintained to each section of the installation in the event of failure involving one transformer high voltage feeder.

15.8   A typical Nucleus development may have two equally rated transformer units installed in a centrally sited sub-station as the most economical arrangement. Other arrangements in an HCP may involve a larger number of sub-station compact transformers fed from the ring main system. The aim should be to cover as much distribution as is practicable with high voltage cables. Figures 3 to 5 show typical distribution circuits.

15.9   With the cyclic load pattern normally experienced in HCPs, and taking into consideration capital costs, depreciation, copper and iron losses, it may be economic to overload transformers for short periods. This is applicable only as a temporary measure when the loading is known accurately. CP1010 'Loading guide to transformers' gives guidance for oil immersed transformers.

Size of transformers

15.10   On a cost per unit kVA basis, the cost of transformers varies inversely as the capacity increases up to 500 kVA, then tends to become more directly proportional. For HCP applications, the most useful size of transformer is that having a capacity of 500 kVA. In large, compact HCPs it may be more economical to raise the maximum capacity to 800 kVA. In general it is desirable to limit the power rating to restrict the fault current level at the low voltage installation and also reduce the extent of interruption of supply in the event of a failure involving one of the transformers.

Transformer winding terminations

15.11   The arrangement of the end terminals of each of the three winding phases in both the HV and LV sides of a transformer determines the angle of displacement or phase shift in the LV output phase voltage relative to the HV input phase voltage.

15.12   The arrangement of the end terminals of each of the three-phase windings in both the HV and LV sides determines the phase shift in the LV output phase voltage by the following nomenclature:

a.   HV   phase 1 (R) – $A_1 \rightarrow A_2$;
        phase 2 (Y) – $B_1 \rightarrow B_2$;
        phase 3 (B) – $C_1 \rightarrow B_2$;

b.   LV   phase 1 (r) – $a_1 \rightarrow a_2$;
        phase 2 (y) – $b_1 \rightarrow b_2$;
        phase 3 (b) – $c_1 \rightarrow c_2$.

15.13   Vectorially, the three-phase HV vectors are shown in a delta or star arrangement. The HV phase 1 (R) vector is shown vertical. The LV phase 1 (r) vector, with respect to the (R) vector, is angled in a separate delta or star arrangement. The associated Y, B and y, b vectors assume a 120° phase shift.

15.14 Details for the construction of vector configurations for transformers are given in BS171:Part 4 (IEC76:Part 4) – 'Specification for tappings and connections'.

15.15 A standard type of transformer terminal configuration is the delta-star, Dy11 connection. This represents the HV phase vector leading by +30° relative to the corresponding LV vector. Dy11 is the standard winding connection configuration for 11,000/433 V, three-phase transformers, supplying power from the regional electricity company (REC) to HCPs.

15.16 Transformers are not normally paralleled at the LV side, owing to the higher maximum prospective fault current at the LV side.

Mineral oil immersed transformers

15.17 The Electricity Association document EA35-1 aims to standardise and rationalise with a view to saving costs. Transformers complying with this standard will be suitable for healthcare premises applications where the use of mineral oil-cooled transformers is considered appropriate. EA35-1 is based upon BS171 type ONAN. The standard sizes appropriate to HCP use are 11 kV/433 V, Dy11, three-phase rated at 315, 500 and 800 kVA, with off-load tap changing facilities to allow ±2.5% and ±5% variation at 75°C.

15.18 The figures for mineral oil-cooled transformers quoted in Table 7 are specified in EA Std 35-1.

15.19 Sealed or free breathing and sub-station compact transformers are available at suitable ratings. Pressure and temperature actuated relays are provided with sealed tank transformers. Pipe connected silica-gel absorption filters and temperature actuated relays are provided with free breathing transformers.

Dry type transformers

15.20 Both dry types of air-cooled transformers are established designs:

a. the open wound type transformer has class "200" insulation (old class "C"). In this transformer the open construction of the winding and the nature of the insulating material used make it prone to small free emissions of halogen gases when subjected to fire. BS2757 refers;

b. the epoxy resin-cast type wound transformer may be less expensive. It contains both class "H" and class "F" insulations. These comprise a dense, epoxy-resin encapsulated HV winding having excellent insulation to withstand over-voltage surges. When subjected to fire, the emission of halogen gases from the fire-retardant insulation is minimal owing to the dense, sealed construction provided by the epoxy-resin casting or mixed epoxy-resin and silica/glass fibre insulation encapsulating the winding assembly;

c. the aluminium foil conductor is preferred to the copper foil conductor in the epoxy-resin cast of the transformer HV windings. Aluminium has a more compatible expansion/contraction characteristic in maintaining a tight void-free contact between the epoxy resin and the transformer winding conductor during the liquid epoxy resin encapsulating pour and heat curing process.

15.21 In aluminium-wound transformers the rate of temperature change with respect to load change is not as rapid as in a similar copper-wound transformer. This results in an overall reduction in relative mechanical movement between the conductors and the epoxy-resin insulation, and in the formation of winding void spaces and sources of voltage stress.

In the event of transformers being connected in parallel, it is essential that the nomenclature of connections of each transformer is identical, that is, Dy 11 in parallel with Dy 11. A variation in the clock numerical value would mean the circulation of a large current between both transformers and failure to operate, due to overcurrent and overheating to both sets of windings. In all cases the LV winding must be star connected to permit the connection of the star point to the main earth system.

15.22   Aluminium or copper foils are used equally in the LV winding. The LV winding insulation is impregnated with epoxy resin, sealed, then heat cured to harden. Cooling ducts are placed axially in the LV winding to provide natural or forced air-cooling paths.

15.23   The LV winding is assembled nearest to the iron core and concentric with the HV winding assembly. The foil (that is roll) construction of the windings eliminates axial winding stresses that are present in strip windings under fault conditions.

15.24   Both types of transformer can be enclosed in indoor, low-priced, open ventilated, door interlocked steel cubicles, and stand next to the 415 V switchboard where required. Forced-air ventilation, automatically controlled by winding hot spot sensors, can be provided, or provision made for it in the initial core frame construction. This may give an intermittent load increase up to 130% rating.

15.25   The open type winding requires a clean, dust-free environment, but the resin cast type may operate, where specified with sealed terminations, in a dusty or heavily polluted environment.

15.26   Generally, the cast epoxy resin is considered a more suitable transformer for building services requirements. The open type is used more for industrial switchroom uses and is treated now as a special order by manufacturers, which reflects in higher manufacturing cost and ex-works prices.

15.27   Dry type transformers are noisier in operation than liquid-cooled transformers, therefore building acoustic insulation may be required to avoid noise nuisance and sound resonance. Transformers should conform to the noise level requirements of BS6056.

15.28   If not screened with an adequate steel enclosure, the magnetic field produced by transformer currents flowing in the cable works and bus-bars can cause interference to data equipment and eliminate disk data within the building.

Synthetic fluid immersed transformers

15.29   The mineral oil cooling in indoor transformers constitutes an unacceptable fire risk. Synthetic insulating fluids Formel (NF), Midal, silicon and others have been available for a long time in limited manufacture. Formel NF and mineral insulating oil must not be mixed or interchanged. Midal can be added to mineral oil if required without affecting the transformer rating. A maximum of 10% silicon may be added to mineral oil.

Askarel

15.30   Askarel is a banned non-flammable fluid containing polychlorinated biphenyls (PCBs). It is compatible with transformer class A insulation. It was used in the manufacture of transformers to BS171 and complied with the Electricity Association document ESI 35-11 (withdrawn). The fluid askarel PCB was banned from use in 1984. Transformers and power factor correction capacitors and other equipment containing askarel which were manufactured before 1984 can remain in service, but must be phased out when feasible.

15.31   Askarel does not evaporate at normal air temperature, is carcinogenic, and is persistent in the food chain. Askarel is not easily replaced in existing transformers by mineral oil. It can be done, but is a costly and tedious operation requiring strict health and environmental controls to reduce the safe level of concentration by dilution and replacement techniques, and is unlikely to lead to a satisfactory conclusion.

Formel NF

15.32   The synthetic insulating fluid Formel NF is non-flammable. It contains basically 67% perchloroethylene (PERC) and 33% chlorofluorocarbon (CFC) and will not ignite when subjected to a high energy electric arc or fire. It is volatile and can be smelled below the working long-term exposure limit (LTEL) of 50 ppm at normal temperatures, and should be well contained, as leakages will evaporate quickly. High concentrations can have short-term narcotic affects. The electrical characteristics of Formel NF are similar to mineral oil. The thermal stability is absolute and heat transfer is superior. Formel NF-cooled transformers have a smaller volume/power ratio than mineral oil, Midal or silicon-cooled transformers. Electricity Association document 35–14 refers.

15.33   There are no known by-products produced (1992) when NF is subjected to heat or adverse ambient conditions that might constitute a health hazard. Containment must be carefully controlled. Recovery and reprocessing of Formel NF from redundant transformers is part of the manufacturer's service.

15.34   Because of the CFC content, the use of Formel NF will be regulated by the Montreal Protocol 1990 relating to ozone layer-depleting chemicals.

Midal fluid

15.35   The synthetic insulating fluid "Midal 7131" has the chemical name pentaerythritol ester. It is an almost non-volatile, straw-coloured liquid with a faint sweet smell. Midal is flammable, as it can be ignited by high energy electrical arcs and by external heat. The flashpoint temperature is 257°C. Water mist, foam, CO_2 and dry powder can be used to fight any fires.

15.36   Spillage residues may be removed with detergent solutions and dry sand. It is a non-irritant to the eyes and skin. Protective coveralls and impervious gloves should be used when handling Midal, as required with mineral insulating oil. No breathing apparatus is required to remove spillages. Waste disposal should only be carried out to environmental, local and statutory regulations.

15.37   Environmentally, Midal has no known toxic or long-term health problems to man, fauna or plant life.

Silicon fluid

15.38   The synthetic insulating fluid "Silicon 561" is from the chemical family polydimethyl siloxane (PDMS) as used in anti-perspirants, hair sprays, body implants and food preparations. It is a non-volatile (below 230°C) clear fluid with a slight smell.

15.39   Silicon is flammable, as it can be ignited by high energy electrical arcs and by external heat. The flashpoint temperature is 300°. The total heat release from Silicon 561 is small compared with mineral insulating oil during combustion, releasing silica ash, CO, CO_2 and trace quantities of H_2 and O_2. No protective clothing except coveralls and safety glasses, is required when handling Silicon 561. Breathing apparatus is not required to remove spillages.

15.40   Environmentally, Silicon 561 has no known related problems to man. It is non-biodegradable and does not mix with water. Any releases to the environment should be mixed with sand. It should be handled as mineral insulating oil.

15.41   Disposal should be carried out to environmental, local and statutory regulations.

Developments in synthetic fluids

15.42   Further developments are taking place in synthetic insulating fluids which are more environmentally acceptable for use in non-flammable transformers. In the course of a few years, these may provide an alternative to the existing synthetic insulating fluids.

Synthetic fluid containment

15.43   Transformers containing synthetic insulating fluid must be of the sealed tank type, the tank cover being welded to the tank. The tank is filled when under a partial vacuum at ambient temperature. The gas vapour blanket over the liquid contains low partial pressure air or nitrogen.

15.44   Fittings will be as for mineral oil transformers:

a.   a pressure relief valve is required instead of a breather;

b.   a lockable drain valve without a sampling device is required instead of a combined drain plug and sampling device.

15.45   A pressure/trip switch is required to monitor transformer tank vapour pressure for tank leakage while on load, when Formel NF is the coolant.

15.46   Synthetic insulating fluid-filled transformers are delivered as sealed units from which there should be no leakage of fluid under normal conditions. The transformer should, however, be examined when received for any leakage or spillage that may have occurred during transportation. Following installation, periodic in-service inspection should be made for leaks. Any leaks should be monitored and reported to the manufacturer for immediate attention. As these transformers are of the sealed type, spare fluid need not be held locally.

15.47   There are some site safety limitations. The transformer can be located indoors in a locked room well ventilated to the atmosphere and close to working areas. If the transformer is located where a major leak would present a hazard to health, a catchment arrangement below a sealed transformer is required in the unlikely event of fluid leakage, for example in the bund wall.

15.48   In the event of a serious spillage, protective clothing must be available for use. For transformers with Formel NF transformer cooling, self-air-breathing sets and eye-shields must also be available.

15.49   Rating and diagram plates should be in accordance with EA35–1. When Formel NF is the transformer coolant liquid, a warning plate 150 mm x 100 mm made of durable and non-corroding material should be fixed in a prominent position adjacent to the rating and connection plates, bearing the following wording:

> **CAUTION**
>
> The insulation fluid in this transformer is Formel NF and contains a mixture of perchloroethylene (PERC) and chlorofluorocarbon (CFC). Great care should be taken to prevent any loss to the environment. In the event of spillage or leakage or the need for disposal of the transformer, consult Health Technical Memorandum 2007 – 'Electrical services: supply and distribution'.

Handling and disposal of askarels containing polychlorinated biphenyls (PCBs) in transformers, power capacitors and fluorescent/discharge luminaire capacitors

General

15.50   Askarels are non-biodegradable and can accumulate in animals, birds, fish and crustaceans, on which they have long-term toxic effects. Assimilation of askarels in sufficient quantity in humans may cause dermatitis, liver damage and jaundice. They are carcinogenic and easily penetrate skin tissue. For this reason their use is now banned as cooling and insulating fluids.

Handling

15.51   Care must be taken to avoid contact to the skin with an askarel, but should it occur, the skin, which is absorbent, must be thoroughly washed with soap and water as soon as possible. Should askarel enter the eyes, wash thoroughly for at least ten minutes and seek medical aid. Should askarel enter the mouth or stomach, medical aid must be obtained immediately. Always confirm that old equipment in service, if not marked as containing an askarel, does not contain the liquid.

15.52   Full protective clothing must be worn when handling an askarel, which should only be undertaken in a well-ventilated atmosphere. The clothing should be impervious overalls; rubber or neoprene are not suitable. Full-face respirators with head covering should be used, with approved gauntlets for the hands to BS2091. Askarel is not a volatile fluid at normal temperature and pressure.

Disposal

15.53   Disposal of an askarel must be in accordance with the Control of Pollution (Special Waste) Regulations 1980 SI 1980/1709. Askarel spillage must be disposed of by immediately notifying the appropriate local waste disposal authority and an approved specialist firm, who will, where practicable, arrange for disposal. Alternatively, by arrangement with the firm concerned, it should be delivered to them in non-leaking drums clearly labelled with their contents.

The Control of Pollution (Special Waste) Regulations (Northern Ireland) 1981, SR 252/1981

Disposal of askarel-cooled equipment

15.54   Apparatus which is to be scrapped must first be drained and the fluid disposed of as above. This is particularly important if apparatus is to be sold direct to a scrap merchant. The disposal of any fluid waste containing more than 50 ppm askarels PCB is subject to statutory control.

15.55   Alternatively, arrangements may be made for filled apparatus to be sent to an approved specialist disposal firm. In such cases written confirmation and prior approval must be obtained from the local environmental health waste disposal authority and the disposal firm, that they are aware that the apparatus is askarel-cooled and that they will dispose of the fluid by high-temperature incineration.

Specialist advice

15.56   Approved specialist advice and information can be obtained from the area office of the Health and Safety Executive, in leaflet IND(G)34L, and from the Department of the Environment booklet 'Waste Management Paper No 6 – Polychlorinated Biphenyl (PCB) Wastes' (HMSO – ISBN 0 11 751000 9). A list of approved specialist firms can be obtained from the Health and Safety Executive.

Handling and disposal of Formel NF containing 67% perchloroethylene (PERC) and 33% chlorofluorocarbon (CFC) used in transformers and power capacitors

General

15.57   Formel NF is toxicologically acceptable in its manufacture, use, maintenance and disposal scenarios. It is capable of being recycled and purified for re-use. PERC and CFC have been in general use for a long time in the dry-cleaning, manufacturing and laundering processes and as refrigerant gases. At present, substitutes are being sought and tested. There are no known carcinogenic or toxic effects that long-term exposure will cause.

15.58   Environmentally, PERC has been found in drinking water tables and is coming under increasing scrutiny. CFC is identified as contributory to atmospheric ozone-layer decay. The use of CFC chemicals in domestic products such as aerosols and refrigerators is becoming unacceptable.

Handling

15.59   Care must be taken to avoid contact of the skin with Formel NF but should it occur, the skin, which is absorbent, must be thoroughly washed with soap and water as soon as possible. Should Formel NF enter the eyes, wash thoroughly for at least ten minutes and seek medical aid. Should Formel NF enter the mouth or stomach, medical aid must be obtained immediately.

15.60   Formel NF is a non-flammable, colourless liquid with a perceptible odour. It does not mix with water and is 1.6 times heavier than water. The characteristics associated with Formel NF are:

a.   it is volatile at normal temperature and pressure;

b.   the vapour is invisible and heavier than air;

c.   it spreads as a vapour at ground level;

d.   it decomposes in fire giving off a non-toxic irritant fume;

e.   the vapour is an irritant to the eyes;

f.   it has a narcotic effect;

g.   it produces delayed symptoms which may develop after a lapse of a few hours.

15.61   Full protective clothing must be worn when handling Formel NF, which should then only take place in a well-ventilated atmosphere. All clothing, gloves and boots worn must be impermeable to Formel NF, for example by being polythene covered. Full face self-air-breathing sets must be worn in concentrations at or above a short-term exposure limit (STEL) of 10 mins at 150 ppm, and a long-term exposure limit (LTEL) of 8 hours at 50 ppm (subject to Health and Safety Executive revision). All vapour concentration levels must be continuously recorded using an approved halocarbon monitoring instrument. Mechanical ventilation to atmosphere must be provided if natural ventilation is not adequate to reduce area exposure levels.

Disposal of Formel NF

15.62   Disposal of Formel NF must be in accordance with the Control of Pollution (Special Waste) Regulations 1980 SI 1980/1709. A large spillage must be disposed of immediately. Leakage into drainage systems or vegetation must be notified immediately to the local waste disposal authority.

15.63   After recovery, Formel NF should be kept in sealed steel drums. Spillage should be recovered through a vacuum suction hose connected to a steel drum, which is evacuated by a vapour pump exhausting to atmosphere outside the enclosure area. All residues should be recovered by using dry sand, earth or sawdust as the absorbing medium, and put into polythene bags for later burning off at high temperatures at waste disposal centres suitably equipped with approved incinerators.

Disposal of Formel NF-cooled apparatus

15.64   The local waste disposal authority must be notified and transport approval obtained if moved. The manufacturer should be requested to recover the Formel NF for recycling.

15.65   Current regulations (1992) permit, after draining, for the apparatus to be opened to the atmosphere allowing the residual Formel NF to evaporate.

Specialist advice

15.66   Information should be sought primarily from the Health and Safety Executive for written guidance and from the Department of the Environment for detailed literature. The manufacturer has detailed information regarding the chemical and operating characteristics of Formel NF.

16.0 Cables

High voltage cables

Types of cable

Paragraphs 16.48 to 16.60 refer

16.1   For internal tunnel or external cable trench routes, on trays, in conduits, ducts or laid directly in the ground, the following common types of cable are in general use:

a.   xlpe insulated, copper conductors, steel wire (sw) armoured, pvc outer sheath to BS6622, up to 33 kV;

b.   epr insulated, copper conductors sw armoured, pvc outer sheath to BS6622, up to 33 kV;

c.   pvc insulated, copper conductors, sw armoured with pvc outer sheath to BS6346, up to 3.3 kV only;

d.   paper insulated lead covered (pilc) copper or aluminium conductors with or without armour, with pvc outer sheath.

16.2   Where required, single core cable should be provided with aluminium tape or wire (aw) armour and a copper tape screen. The cable should be glanded at non-magnetic gland plates. An insulated terminating gland may be necessary on long cable routes using armoured single core cables to prevent induced circulating current flowing through the armour, which will reduce the cable rating or the effectiveness of E/F protection where a current transformer is placed in the glanded length of cable.

16.3   The open circuit induced voltage between the armour and earth should not exceed 25 volts when full load current flows in the cable, and where insulated terminating glands are used.

16.4   Inside buildings, the laying of single core three-phase cables in trefoil or enclosure in steel ducting or conduit may be required to reduce magnetic field-induced interference to medical and data processing equipment.

Comparisons

16.5   The choice of cable will be largely influenced by cost comparisons. The cost saving with epr/pvc/xlpe types of cables has resulted in their increasing use and is a very significant factor with larger schemes.

16.6   Pvc and xlpe insulations are of comparable price. The lower operating temperature limitation of pvc requires the cable sizes to be larger than are required for xlpe, providing there is not a volt drop criterion.

16.7   Pvc cable has a restricted HV range, limited to 3.3 kV.

16.8   Epr insulation offers advantages over xlpe in certain circumstances. It is more flexible, making it easier to install in difficult situations and more appropriate where it may be subject to movement or flexing in use, that is, as a trailing cable. It also offers greater resistance to water penetration when direct buried, and better fire-resistance performance. On the negative side, epr is 5–10% greater in cost than xlpe cable.

Maximum temperature and fault current ratings

16.9   All cable must be capable of satisfactorily withstanding the maximum prospective fault current (mpfc) of the system for the period of time needed for the fault to be cleared by the protection equipment. The thermal damage to equipment under fault conditions increases as the square of the fault current multiplied by time, and this is a very important factor where time discriminating protection is employed.

16.10   The 1-second mpfc current ratings of high voltage cables are given in the cable manufacturers' brochures. Appropriate design data is also given for cable laying, which should include at full load rating, correction factors for temperature variations, grouping and spacing of cables; and for cables in free air, confined spaces or buried directly or in ducts, also minimum bending radii and general handling of cables during installation.

16.11   As there is no lead or aluminium sheath normally provided in pvc, epr or xlpe insulated cable, a copper tape is wound around the conductor insulation to act as a screen and to provide a suitably low resistance and earth return path for HV cable protection earth fault current. The earth fault current rating of this screen must be adequate to exceed the elapsed time delay before the protection relay and the circuit breaker operate.

16.12   Table 8 gives an example of the recommended minimum cable sizes for various fault current levels and maximum fault current duration times. The cable sizes for both the pvc insulated cables up to 3.3 kV are based on the assumption of an initial conductor temperature of 70°C and a maximum conductor temperature not exceeding 160°C to BS6004 and BS6346.

Fault duration(s)	0.2	0.3	0.5	1.0	1.5	2	3
				kA			
Area 50 mm^2	15.2	12.4	9.6	6.8	5.5	4.8	3.9
Area 70 mm^2	21.9	17.8	13.8	9.8	8.0	6.9	5.6
Area 95 mm^2	29.7	24.2	18.8	13.3	10.8	9.4	7.6

Table 8   Recommended minimum cable sizes for various fault currents and duration for 11 kV, 3 core copper conductor, xlpe, epr insulated, single wire armoured cables (figures in mpfc, kA)

16.13   The cable ratings are identical for the xlpe and epr insulated cables up to 33 kV and are based on the assumption of an initial conductor temperature of 90°C and a maximum conductor temperature not exceeding 250°C to BS6622.

16.14   The xlpe cable has a lower extended emergency overload current temperature limit of 105°C. This lower temperature is to limit the effects of cable radial and axial expansion. The equivalent epr cable limiting temperature is 130°C.

Paper insulated lead covered cables

16.15   Paper insulated lead covered (pilc) cables are no longer considered a first choice in the installation of HV cables up to 11 kV. More suitable and practical alternatives are available. The additional cost and work involved on site have made their installation uneconomic. At higher voltages, 33 kV and above, they are used in selected installations. The paper insulation is superior and the overall dimensions are less than for xlpe or epr insulation.

16.16   The maximum operating temperature of the copper conductor, or initial temperature for fault calculations in paper insulated lead covered cables, is limited to 65°C and a maximum conductor fault temperature of 160°C, that is, they are very similar to pvc insulation requirements.

16.17   Pilc use has been superseded by xlpe, epr and pvc. Pilc can only be supplied at extra cost, in minimum lengths (say 250 m). It is no longer supplied ex-stock by manufacturers. In an extreme case of mains-borne electromagnetic interference, this type of cable may offer a solution.

16.18   A lead sheathed cable requires a lead wiped seal at the gland, sealed by hot bitumen compound poured into the cable box. This greatly increases the cost of installation for terminating and jointing. Compression glands for pilc entries into a cable box are not recommended by leading manufacturers, on safety grounds.

Cable installation

16.19   Cables should be joint-free as far as is practicable. Joints can be avoided if specified measured cable route lengths on a cable drum are provided by the cable manufacturer.

16.20   Where joints are necessary they should be made in accordance with the codes of practice provided by manufacturers of high voltage joints, or as applicable, by the Electricity Association – 'Engineering recommendations for pilc cable', document C34.

16.21   Across any armoured joint the cable screen and conductor electrical resistance should not exceed that of an equivalent length of cable with complete armouring.

16.22   For short cable runs in protected vermin-free conduits or accessible covered steel ducts (for example in sub-stations), armoured cables will not be required.

16.23   Armoured protection must be provided where cables may be subject to mechanical damage during installation. Cables having single wire armouring should then be used to avoid any possibility of damage to insulation and outer sheath.

16.24   Inside buildings, and in areas where the presence of toxic hydrochloric acid halogen fumes would be unacceptable in fire conditions, the use of fire-retardant, halogen-free, low smoke-emitting, xlpe insulated cables and bedding, with inner sleeve and outer sheath to BS6724, is advised.

16.25   For external runs, single wire steel armoured, pvc outer sheathed cables are preferred. Where cables are subjected to excessive stresses, for example where land subsidence is likely, double wire steel armouring should be specified.

16.26   Epr cable should be used in preference to xlpe cable in waterlogged ground.

Cable glands and terminations

16.27   HV cable glands must be rated above the prospective fault current of the system to which they are assembled. The glands should have integral earth lugs to which equibonding copper strip connects to the main copper earth bar.

16.28   If required, the cable armour secured at the cable gland could be isolated or separated from the equipment by an island type insulating gland.

16.29   HV cable boxes should be made of fabricated steel and terminations, air insulated up to 11 kV. Spacing between the terminals must conform to BS4999/145 or IEC standards requirements for the rated voltage.

16.30   All HV terminations and terminating cable tails should also be encapsulated in heat shrinkable, voltage graded plastic insulation, approved and guaranteed by a reputable manufacturer for the rated voltage.

16.31   Steel cable boxes for the high voltage terminations of rotating machines should be provided with an aluminium foil explosion diaphragm, and as a safety precaution, the boxes preferably orientated to face a nearby reinforced concrete vertical surface or 200 mm brick wall. A splash protected breather hole with an external replaceable silica gel dryer with screwed insert should be provided to prevent the accumulation of condensed water vapour within the cable box.

16.32   All cables should be marked and terminated in an approved manner to indicate phases. The far and near phase cable ends must be checked by continuity meter to confirm identical phase markings.

16.33   The oversheath of HV cable, exposed between gland and floor, should be mechanically protected from in-situ damage.

Low voltage distribution cables

General types of cable

16.34   For distribution in tunnels, conduits, ducts or laid directly in the ground, the following common types are in general use:

   a. pvc insulated, copper conductors, sw armoured with pvc outer sheath to BS6346;

   b. xlpe insulated, copper conductors, sw armoured with pvc outer sheath;

   c. xlpe insulated copper conductors, sw armoured with low-smoke, halogen-free bedding and outer sheath to BS6724;

   d. mineral insulated, copper sheathed (mims) heavy-duty, having copper conductors and sheathed with pvc outer covering to BS6207 and tested to BS6387;

   e. lapped mica-glass tape or silicon rubber insulated copper conductor, sw armoured or non-armoured and low-smoke halogen-free outer sheath and bedding to BS6724 and tested to BS6387 for the temperature level required.

Choice of cables

16.35   Choice will be influenced by size, method of installation and number of terminations. The maximum cable terminations available in transformer or circuit breaker LV cable boxes are normally two cable cores per phase. Three cores or more will require precise specification.

16.36   The use of aluminium conductors in preference to copper conductors is not practical nor economical. Aluminium cables as rated are larger, require greater space, are difficult to lay, and require larger glands and cable lugs for terminations.

16.37 For general cable work, pvc, xlpe or elastomeric insulated cables greatly simplify installation where terminating and jointing is required, compared to mineral insulated cable.

16.38 There is no metallic conducting screen with pvc, elastomeric or xlpe LV insulated cable. Therefore, special attention is necessary to ensure that the wire armouring is earthed at all the cable gland connections. The gland should be correctly rated for the sub-circuit prospective fault current.

16.39 Insulated type glands to BS6121 should be used on all incoming armoured power cables feeding data equipment. This would remove parasitic earths and reduce electromagnetic interference to the data equipment.

Joints

16.40 Straight-through and tee joints should not be used unless economically unavoidable. In any cable, the armoured joint's electrical resistance should not exceed that of an equivalent length of unjointed armoured cable.

16.41 Single core cable armour must be non-magnetic wire or tape.

16.42 When power cables are cut during installation, the ends should be sealed to prevent moisture penetration (to be carried out in the manner recommended by the manufacturer).

16.43 Low voltage joints should be made in accordance with the cable manufacturer's recommendations.

Minimum bending radii and supports for cables

16.44 The minimum internal bending radii for cables should not be less than the value for that type of cable given in the appropriate British Standard, the IEE Wiring Regulations or manufacturer's brochure.

16.45 If the minimum radius is too small, it must not be used when end-pulling cables through ducts or around conduit radial bends.

16.46 Cables should be adequately supported throughout the route length. The spacing between points of support should be within the values given in the IEE Wiring Regulations and manufacturer's recommendations.

16.47 Cable plastics should not be exposed to direct sunlight without sun shade protection. Some cable plastic sheath and insulation may contain unsuitable matrix filler material. This may permit premature embrittlement or ageing of the plastic in sunlight. The cable manufacturer should be consulted where cables are subject to exposed environments.

Insulating materials in cables

General

16.48 Most modern cables up to 11 kV, in general applications, use polymeric insulation and sheathing, although some Regional Electricity Companies (RECs) may still use paper-insulated cables for high voltage distribution. There are two broad classes of polymeric insulation: thermoplastic and elastomeric (or thermosetting).

Thermoplastic materials

16.49   Thermoplastic materials are insulating materials which do not return to their original state after excessive deformation. In general they offer excellent electrical properties with low losses and low permittivity. Thermoplastics used in cables include polyvinyl chloride (pvc), polyethylene and polypropylene.

Polyvinyl chloride

16.50   Polyvinyl chloride (pvc) is the material most widely used for cable insulation and sheaths at low voltages up to 3.3 kV. It offers good resistance to chemical and mechanical damage. General-purpose pvc is suitable for a maximum conductor temperature of 70°C. Below 0°C it tends to harden but recovers flexibility when it returns to normal ambient temperatures. Pvc offers flame-retardant qualities but emits dense acrid smoke and toxic fumes in a fire.

Polyethylene

16.51   Polyethylene offers superior electrical properties and water resistance and is the preferred insulant for radio frequency cables, but has not found widespread use for power cables where its thermoplastic properties make it a less suitable material than cross-linked polyethylene (xlpe).

Fluorocarbon tapes and extrusions

16.52   Materials such as polytetrafluoroethylene (ptfe), fluorinated ethylene propylene (fep), ethylene tetrafluoroethylene and polyamide/fep tapes are used for high performance cables in the aircraft and other industries. They offer excellent electrical properties, high operating temperatures, resistance to chemical attack, and a thinner wall permits lower weight.

Elastomeric materials

16.53   Elastomeric (or thermoset) materials return to their original shape and dimensions after deformation. They tend to have a wider operational temperature range and superior mechanical properties compared with general-purpose thermoplastic materials. This makes them particularly suited to cable sheathing applications, especially in arduous environments. Elastomeric materials suitable for cable applications include ethylene propylene rubber (epr), cross-linked polyethylene (xlpe), ethylene vinyl acetate, natural rubber, silicon rubber, chlorosulphonated polyethylene, chlorinated polyethylene and polychloroprene.

Ethylene propylene rubber

16.54   Ethylene propylene rubber (epr) is widely used for insulation and some sheathing, especially for distribution cables. It offers the flexibility of natural rubber but with higher operating temperatures (90°). It is also easier to strip. Hard grade epr is also available.

Cross-linked polyethylene

16.55   Cross-linked polyethylene (xlpe) is well-established at higher voltages and is frequently preferred to epr or hepr on a cost basis. It is less flexible than epr and even pvc but offers a higher operating temperature (90°C) than pvc, which means that under certain conditions the current rating of the cables may be increased by 15-20%. This can be a particular advantage in the tropics. Significantly higher symmetrical short-circuit ratings are also possible corresponding to a conductor temperature of 250°C during fault conditions. This is compared with 150°C for pvc cables. Xlpe will ignite and burn readily but has low smoke and fume emission characteristics.

Ethylene vinyl acetate

16.56   Ethylene vinyl acetate forms the basis of most modern low-smoke zero-halogen cable sheath materials. Many of its properties are similar to those of epr although resistance to oil, water and abrasion are not as good as chlorosulphonated polyethylene and polychloroprene.

Silicon rubber

16.57   Silicon rubber is used as an insulation and offers a conductor with higher operating temperature (150°C continuous) than natural rubber or ethylene vinyl acetate. When burned, silicon rubber is converted to a silicon dioxide ash which has similar electrical qualities and volume to the original material; this property is exploited in some modern fire-resisting cables.

Chlorosulphonated polyethylene

16.58   Chlorosulphonated polyethylene is a tough, heat-resistant and flame-retardant synthetic rubber which makes an excellent sheathing material for arduous environments. Epr insulation with chlorosulphonated polyethylene oversheath is a popular choice for marine and offshore applications.

Chlorinated polyethylene

16.59   Chlorinated polyethylene offers similar properties to chlorosulphonated polyethylene, for which it is frequently used as an alternative.

Polychloroprene

16.60   Polychloroprene is an oil-resistant and flame-retardant synthetic rubber with high resistance to abrasion. It is ideal for arduous conditions such as in mines and quarries. Heat resistance is inferior to chlorosulphonated polyethylene and chlorinated polyethylene.

17.0 Earthing

Power systems

Generators

17.1   Where 415 V, three-phase emergency generators are installed, a separate earth rod system must be provided. LV generators must be solidly earthed. This earth rod system may be interconnected to the main earth system.

17.2   For island operation, only one parallel LV generator should be solidly earthed. In a multi-generator island system, each generator neutral should be connected separately into an interlocked neutral switchboard. If a connection is required between the earthed neutral and the main earth system, this should be done by an interconnected isolating switch interlocked with the circuit breaker of the incoming REC supply transformer.

17.3   Where HV or LV generators run in parallel, isolated from or synchronised to the REC supply, isolating switching devices must be provided in the star-point neutrals to ensure that only **one** earth connection is possible to the main earth system. HTM 2011 – 'Emergency electrical services' refers.

17.4   HV generators may be earthed by a metal or liquid resistance to restrict generator fault current to a full load current value. Suitable overcurrent and earth fault current protection must be provided at each generator circuit breaker. The REC guidance and requirements must be sought at the design stage of the project.

Earth electrodes

17.5   Earth electrodes for providing the main earth system or ground impedance to the point of supply, should be buried in the ground as near as is practicable to the sub-station or main distribution centre. This should not be less than 3 m from the base of the building, telecommunication or data cables. The extent and the number of rods in the electrode system will depend on the nature of soil resistivity. The latter can vary from summer to winter, and depending on site development.

17.6   A typical electrode would consist of steel cored copper rods 12 mm or 15 mm in diameter, up to 3.6 m long, in 1.2 m lengths. Where more than one rod is required the rods should be spaced apart by a distance at least equal to the length of each rod, in parallel, in two connected but separate groups.

17.7   A low impedance to earth of, say, 2 ohms resistance will permit rapid protection operation and a low touch potential to earth faults. Surface current density "J" of earth electrodes of less than 40 amps/m^2 is required. During a fault, current density increases, hence ground dry-out should be avoided. For an earth electrode, maximum fault current density is typically:

$$J = 10^3 \frac{[57.7]}{[rho]t} \text{ amps/m}^2$$

where t = sec, rho = resistivity ohm × m.

BS7430 'Code of practice for earthing' refers.

The Regional Electricity Company (REC), where their supply is LV, will provide a main earth terminal for use by the HCP for its electrical system. If the intake is at HV, a neutral-star point connection must be made at each transformer LV winding to the main earths.

17.8   Initially, it is recommended that one electrode be installed and the resistance of the ground measured as described in HTM 2007 'Validation and verification'. Provided the rods are spaced apart as stated above, the overall ground impedance will be approximately equal to the impedance of one rod divided by the number of rods employed. In this way the minimum number of rods required to achieve a specific impedance can be determined. The impedance of the final electrode system should be verified by an earth resistance test.

17.9   In hard or rocky terrain, electrodes may have to be inserted into pre-bored holes that have been made porous by explosive. The annular space between rod and hole is filled with a conducting mud slurry commercially known as "bentonite".

17.10   Bare copper strip in a comprehensive lattice can be laid by cross- trenching. This method is difficult to assess at the design stage, and can cause maintenance and excavation problems later, owing to the area of ground utilised by the copper strip.

17.11   Cast-iron plates or pipes can be buried to 3 metre depths. The cast iron parts must be interconnected, and bonded together by copper straps. The connections must be sealed and protected against galvanic corrosion or ground corrosion by the use of a waterproof tape and compound. The use of material as a contact matrix which is high in acidic or alkaline compounds, can accelerate metal corrosion in the cast-iron plates. Such materials are not recommended.

Earth connections

17.12   Terminal connections to earth electrodes should be made in an accessible inspection pit.

17.13   All earth connections must be of the standard split or claw type, of non-zinc bronze with a cable socket. They must be protected from corrosion by a suitable compound impregnated waterproof tape.

17.14   All main earth terminal bars should be protected with pvc sheath where corrosion is likely.

17.15   All directly buried or ducted underground earth cable cores should be stranded and covered with a green pvc outer sheath. The earth cable should be installed at least 0.6 m below ground level, and covered with interlocking cable tiles and route marker tape.

17.16   Where the ground area is very restricted, it may be expedient to bond the structural steel work and reinforcement steel at the lowest level to provide a suitable main earth system. This may cause long-term earth and interference difficulties. Lightning down-conductors must not be linked into such an earth system above ground level.

Main earth bus-bar

17.17   It is usually desirable to have a main earth bus-bar in a secure transformer chamber or low voltage switchroom with connections at approximately 600 mm above the floor level, in an accessible position. The earth bar should be solid copper on insulators and of sufficient length to provide separate identifiable circuit earth group terminals. Typical terminations are as follows:

    a. bare conductors to transformer frames;

    b. bare conductor to high voltage switchgear frame;

    c. bare conductor to low voltage switchgear frame;

d. pvc insulated stranded conductor to sub-station earth electrode(s), run in ducts or directly buried;

e. pvc insulated stranded cable to the low voltage transformer neutral connection, run in ducts or directly buried;

f. emergency generator winding star-point earth connection.

17.18 Earthing cables passing into direct burial, outside concrete trenches or underground ducts should be protected from corrosion by pvc sheathing and be stranded as required.

17.19 Earthing conductors above ground or in dry trenches should be secured to concrete surfaces or steelwork with approved clamps and saddles.

17.20 The minimum size of earthing leads and earth continuity conductors relative to the size of the largest associated circuit conductor should not be less than the value given in the IEE Wiring Regulations.

17.21 Data processing rooms require a short length, low impedance auxiliary electrode cable connection to earth. This directly connected electrode is required to avoid the high impedance earth leakages and noise generated voltage interference produced in interconnected protective conductor connections by other electrical equipment, bonding currents in structural metalwork and electromagnetic radiation.

Figure 13 shows a typical sub-station earthing system. British Standard Code of Practice CP1013 deals with various aspects of earthing.
IEC publication 36A–7–707 – 'Earthing requirements for installation of data processing equipment', and HTM 2014 – 'Abatement of electrical interference' refer.

Lightning protection

British Standards requirements (BS6651:1992)

17.22 Whether or not elaborate lightning protection is justified will depend on the height of the buildings and the location of the HCP. As some areas are more prone to lightning than others, British Standard 6651:1985 – 'Protection of structures against lightning' includes a probability equation which is intended as a guide in determining whether or not a particular building should have lightning protection. Using this equation, it may be found that main HCP buildings (not used for patient accommodation) need not be separately protected. Frequently they may come within the protection zone of nearby taller buildings that are protected.

Lightning protection systems

17.23 A lightning protection system will consist of air terminations, roof conductors, down-conductors, bonds to exposed permanent metal parts of the building, testing points, earth terminations and earth electrodes. The installation should be designed in accordance with BS6651–'Protection of structures against lightning'. Small buildings may not require protection if the BS6651 probability equation indicates a small chance of a lightning strike.

Materials

17.24 Appropriate copper and copper alloys to BS2870 and BS2874 and aluminium alloys to BS2898 are suitable for air terminations, roof conductors and down-conductors.

17.25 Earth terminations and electrodes should be of copper or copper alloys. Steel cored rods may be used for earth electrodes where acidic ground corrosion is not severe, otherwise solid copper should be used. In ground where there is galvanic corrosion due to large quantities of dissimilar buried metals, austenitic stainless steel rods may be necessary.

17.26   The choice of aluminium instead of copper above ground must be balanced against the relative material cost, handling cost and durability. On building surfaces where corrosive stains would be unsightly, lead covered copper conductors may be considered for aesthetic reasons.

17.27   The risk of corrosion is usually greater with aluminium but can be reduced by taking suitable precautions during installation. Aluminium bare conductors may be used in dry areas above ground but should not be used below ground level.

Zone of protection

17.28   For practical purposes, it can be assumed that a lightning conductor will protect the space within the volume of a 45° upright cone when the conductor is at the apex point, or the space outside the circumferential locus of contact described by the surface of a rolling sphere of 20 m radius, at those points where it makes contact with the lightning conductor.

17.29   This must be taken into consideration when providing personnel protection at building exits and entrances containing metalwork structures, and for temporary installations assembled during construction or servicing, that is, scaffolding or cranes.

Aerials

17.30   Special attention should be given to the protection of television and radio aerials. These should be protected by bonding the tubular support of the aerial to the lightning protection system.

Chimneys

17.31   A chimney of non-conducting material, of which the height exceeds 20 m and the overall width of the top exceeds 1.5 m, should have at least two down-conductors equally spaced, bonded by a metal cap or by a conductor around the top of the chimney. The use of two down-leads will allow loop continuity testing of the down-leads. For small chimneys, a single, unjointed conductor can be used. Aluminium may be superior to copper or even lead-coated copper in withstanding exhaust gas corrosion, when used for air terminations on upper parts of particular chimneys.

17.32   Round conductors have, for the same cross-sectional area, a smaller surface area exposed to corrosion. This type of conductor should be used wherever convenient in this type of installation.

Buildings

17.33   20 mm × 3 mm ($\frac{3}{4}$ in × $\frac{1}{8}$ in) or 50 mm diameter annealed copper or aluminium roof conductors are the minimum size. These should be fixed along ridges or around the roof perimeter and interconnected with other conductors run across the roof as necessary, so that no part of the roof is more than 10 m from a conductor.

17.34   Where there is a higher part of the roof such as a tank or plantroom, it should be fitted with a perimeter conductor and joined to the main roof system. Metal edge trims or metal roofing systems, which have sufficient sheet cross-sectional area and a method of jointing which can be made to conform to the requirements of BS6651, may then be used as a roof conductor.

17.35   Roof conductors should be fixed, for example with saddles, at intervals not exceeding 1 m. The fixing should have sufficient clearance around the conductor to allow for water drainage and freedom from contact with mortar, and for any movement due to solar or building expansion and contraction. Special expansion loops will not normally be necessary. In exposed risk areas, the roof conductors should be arranged in a 10 m × 20 m mesh.

17.36   Building structures exceeding 20 m in height are given a separate new approach in BS6651. A 20 m radius rolling sphere is passed around and over the building. Points of the building that are outside the possible contact arc of the rolling sphere surface are considered protected from direct or side lightning strikes.

17.37   Those areas of a building fabric that make surface or point contact with the sphere surface are considered vulnerable. They are unprotected from direct or side lightning strokes and must be given lightning protection at the points of spherical contact with a 20 m × 10 m roof conductor lattice. Buildings up to 20 m in height must be protected in the normal approved manner.

17.38   Lower buildings that lie within the 45° horizontally subtended cone angle of higher conductors, for example that on a chimney or adjacent building, do not need separate protection.

Air terminations

17.39   It is not necessary to provide finials as air terminations. Finials involve additional joints and do not significantly improve the protection afforded by properly installed roof conductors.

17.40   In systems where the conductors are located below tiled roofs, protruding finials are recommended by BS6651.

Exposed metal parts of structures

17.41   All metallic projections such as radio and television aerial masts, chimneys, ducts, vent pipes, or railings on or above the main surface of the roof, should be bonded to parts of the air termination network. Where dissimilar metals are involved, there should be complete waterproof protection of the joint and effective insulation of the conductor, for example by pvc covering, to prevent any possibility of damp contact between dissimilar metals.

17.42   In reinforced concrete structures the steel bars should be interconnected at roof level, and to the earth conductor system below ground level by a pattern of special earth rods.

17.43   All internal steel structures should be bonded to the roof conductors and to the earth conductor system below ground level by a pattern of special earth rods.

17.44   Exposed metal frames of buildings can be used in place of down-conductors, except fire escapes.

17.45   All metal-framed fire escapes, entrance canopies, exits and walkway systems must be bonded to the down-conductors.

Down-conductors

17.46   Down-conductors of 20 mm × 3 mm ($\frac{3}{4}$ in × $\frac{1}{8}$ in) copper or aluminium strip, or 50 mm diameter rod, are the minimum. They should follow the most direct route between air terminations and earth terminations and where practicable should run vertically down the outside of the building.

17.47   Where an external route cannot be followed and it is necessary to run in a segregated vertical duct through the structure, the appropriate requirements of BS6651 should be complied with.

17.48   Down-conductors and fixing saddles should be tight, and spaced at intervals not exceeding 1 m so that the weight is evenly distributed over the fixings, or at lesser intervals according to BS6651 requirements.

Testing joints

17.49   Each down-conductor should have a test joint in a convenient position but where it cannot be interfered with by unauthorised persons.

17.50   No connection other than direct to an earth electrode should be made below the test joint. The test clamp should be made of the same metal as the conductor or an alloy of this metal complying with the appropriate British Standard (BS6651 refers) and should incorporate facilities to enable the test conductor to be readily clamped to the down-conductor and ensure good electrical contact. Clamping screws should not bear directly on the conductors.

17.51   Where only one down-conductor is provided, the connection to the earth electrode can be used for the test point where it is conveniently accessible. The presence of two down-conductors simplifies routine testing of the roof mesh conductor system.

Number of down-conductors

17.52   One down-conductor is satisfactory for buildings having a base area of less than 100 sq m. One additional down-conductor should be provided for every additional 20 m of the roof perimeter up to 20 m height and for every 10 m roof perimeter above 20 m height. Down-conductors should be kept well clear of doorways.

Joints and bonds to earth

17.53   The essential features of satisfactory jointing are:

  a. adequate mating surface area, not less than 50 sq mm;

  b. cleaning of surfaces, for example with wire wool and clean rag;

  c. mating surfaces coated with petroleum jelly or other suitable anti-corrosion compound immediately after cleaning. Special anti-corrosion compounds are available for aluminium joints;

  d. high pressure clamping, for example by means of bolts or rivets between rigid clamping plates, made of a material with an electrochemical potential close to that of the conductor material. With aluminium conductors, heavy cadmium- or zinc-plated steel plates and bolts are suitable;

  e. complete waterproof protection of joints between dissimilar metals extending at least 75 mm along the conductor on each side of the joint, for example an adequate waterproof coating;

  f. silver soldering or chemical brazing between copper surfaces.

17.54   Each down-conductor requires an earth system connected to the lower side of the test joint. The lower the earth resistance, the greater the protection.

17.55   All underground services adjacent to the lightning protection earth termination which have exposed metal in the form of sheath armouring or piping should be bonded as directly as possible to that earth termination at a point above the test joint.

17.56   The lightning earth rods should be inserted 3 m from the building structure but isolated from footpaths or public access areas.

17.57   A single equipotential bonding conductor should interconnect the lightning earth system to the main earth system below ground level.

Data equipment bonding and earthing

17.58   All data transmission and telephone cables should be placed at least 3 m, or as far as is possible, from an earth rod location to minimise the influence of lightning-generated ground step voltage potentials.

17.59   Data processing equipment power input cables, external data and telephone transmission conductors should be protected by surge arresters to attenuate mains or lightning-induced transient surges. The maximum acceptable attenuated or residual transient voltage must be less than twice the input voltage to ensure survival of the data processing electronic equipment and cable.

Earth resistance

17.60   The resistance to earth of the whole of the lightning protection system should not exceed 10 ohms. Where there is more than one down-lead, the resistance of each individual earth termination in ohms should not exceed ten times the number of earth terminations.

17.61   Reducing the resistance to earth below 10 ohms has the advantage of reducing the voltage step gradient around the earth electrode.

Periodic inspection and testing

17.62   Lightning protection systems should be inspected and tested at least annually; BS6651 refers. Tests should confirm that the earth resistance does not exceed 10 ohms and that the continuity of down-conductors and across any joints in the air termination network is satisfactory.

17.63   The protection system should be regularly inspected to ensure that it is mechanically sound and free from excessive corrosion and that no structural alterations have been made that will affect the system.

Records

17.64   Records, including "as installed" drawings showing the conductor and earthing systems together with dates of inspections and details of test results and any alterations, should be supplied with other handing-over documents.

18.0 Cathodic protection

18.1   In situations where corrosion may occur, for example wet ground/iron systems, a protective measure known as "cathodic protection" (CP) can be applied. The principle is to influence the relative electrolytic voltages of two dissimilar metals by artificial means. Corrosion in metals occurs by movement of negative electrons and positive ions. When iron is immersed in water, O_2 ions in the water attach themselves to the Fe ions, forming iron oxide on the iron exposed surface. By bonding more anodic zinc or magnesium to the iron, these metals will corrode more readily than the iron. A further step is to impress auto-controlled +ve dc onto adjacent electrodes (titanium), the -ve dc connected to the iron mass. The electrolytic current flow is adjusted to polarise the iron to a slightly more negative potential relative to its environment. CP can also be applied in the protection of iron reinforced concrete structures above or below ground level. Care must be exercised where impressed CP is installed near any earthed electrode system. The change in local earth potential may introduce substantial CP return ground current flow through the earthed electrodes, thus accelerating their corrosion. BS7361 refers.

Bond protection code:

1. The joint must have a protective finish after the metal-to-metal contact has been established. This will avoid any bridging of the two metal surfaces by a liquid film.

2. The two metals may be joined with exposed bare metal at the joint. The remainder must be given an appropriate protective finish.

3. This combination can only be used where a short life expectancy is tolerated or when the equipment is normally stored and exposed for only short intervals. Protective coatings are mandatory.

Anodic end (most easily corroded)

Group I	Magnesium
Group II	Aluminium, al alloys, zinc, cadmium, galvanised iron
Group III	Carbon steel, iron, lead, tin, tin-lead solder
Group IV	Nickel, chromium, stainless steel, brass
Group V	Copper, silver, gold, platinum, titanium, bronze

Cathodic end (least corroded)

Groups of materials recommended for providing a protective conductor bond where the joint between any two dissimilar metals forms an anode and cathode

Condition of exposure	Anode connection				To cathode
	I	II	III	IV	
Exposed	A	A			
Sheltered	A	A			II
Housed	A	A			
Exposed	C	A	B		
Sheltered	A	B	B		III
Housed	A	B	B		
Exposed	C	A	B	B	
Sheltered	A	A	B	B	IV
Housed	A	B	B	B	
Exposed	C	C	C	A	
Sheltered	A	A	A	B	V
Housed	A	A	B	B	

Table 9   Chemical series ordered by decreasing sensitivity to corrosion

19.0 Power factor improvement

General

19.1 Typical overall power factors in healthcare premises range between 0.85 and 0.95 lagging. Where a maximum demand charge is specified in kVA it may be economic to provide power factor improvement equipment. It may also be economic where the maximum demand tariff charge is specified in kW, or kVA, and where there is an additional tariff charge for a low power factor. The value at which these charges are levied varies from one regional electricity company (REC) to another.

Equipment

19.2 Capacitors used for mains and luminaire power factor improvements should comply with BS1650. Synthetic liquid immersed power factor improvement capacitors should be of the sealed type, fitted with a warning plate similar to that specified in paragraph 15.44 but substituting "capacitor" for "transformer". General guidance on synthetic liquid filled apparatus is given in paragraph 15.29.

19.3 Where capacitors are installed, care should be taken to eliminate the possibility of an overall leading power factor during periods of light load. This operating condition is best achieved by an automatically controlled switching device to eliminate unwanted capacitor generated leading reactive volt-amperes (kVAr).

19.4 Power factor improvement at selected induction motors has the advantage of reducing the voltage drop in the cable supplying the motor. Capacitor(s) may be connected directly to the motor terminals. Generally this will not affect the run-up or normal running of the motor provided the kVAr rating of the capacitor(s) does not exceed 90% of the full load motor kVAr where direct-on-line or rotor resistor starting is employed (85% if star-delta or autotransformer starting is employed). It is advisable to check this with the motor manufacturer. It will not be economic to apply individual improvement to every motor regardless of size.

19.5 Where power factor improvement equipment is used in installations comprising extensive solid state rectification for battery chargers or uninterrupted power supplies (UPS), a range of harmonic voltages may be reflected back into the supply input. To prevent any natural resonance in any harmonic voltages due to input circuit inductance and capacitance, it may be necessary to install an "in-series" inductor to de-tune any harmonic resonance effects or an input filter unit at the rectifier input. Figure 12 can be used as an aid in determining the capacitor kVAr rating required for power factor improvement to specific values. For example, the dotted line on this nomogram shows that for an initial power factor of 0.7 to be improved to 0.97, the required kVAr is 0.77 × kW load; hence, for a 75 kW load the capacitor rating would be 58 kVAr. Although individual loads might have power factors as low as 0.7 lag, typical overall power factors in HCPs should be greater than 0.9 lag.

20.0 Discrimination and fault conditions

Fault calculations

20.1   Figure 19 analyses the actual three-phase fault levels which may be expected in a typical HCP distribution circuit from the regional electricity company intake, to the power socket-outlet of the final sub-circuit. Evaluation of these sub-circuit fault levels is determined for the five stages up to each switching device or fuse, as shown in Figure 19 and by the following examples, commencing with nominated base values:

given: base values = 1 MVA and 415 V

then: base impedance $(Zb) = \dfrac{\text{voltage base}^2}{\text{MVA base}} = \dfrac{V_b^2}{\text{MVA}_b}$

$\therefore Zb = \dfrac{415^2}{10^6} = 0.172225$ ohms.

From Fig 19, stage 1 cable phase impedance at the 11 kV circuit breaker, as given, is: $Z_1 = 0.00156$ ohms.

20.2   This impedance (or pu) value for stage 1 of the supply must be obtained in practice from the regional electricity company. Then, cable base impedance Z_{cb} in per unit value, at the 11 kV circuit breaker:

$Z_{cb} = \dfrac{Z_1}{Z_b} = \dfrac{0.00156}{0.172225} = 0.009$ pu

and as a cumulative percentage $= 0.009 \times \dfrac{100}{1} = 0.9\%$

$\therefore$ Actual fault current level $= \dfrac{\text{MVA}_b}{Zcb} = \dfrac{10^6}{0.009}$

$= 111.11$ MVA

fault current $= \dfrac{111.11 \times 10^6}{\sqrt{3} \times 415} = 154.6$ kA

20.3   Likewise for the 500 kVA transformer, MVA_t with given impedance Z_t of 4% or 0.04 pu, and stage 2 cable phase impedance Z_c of 0.001 ohm:

a.   transformer base impedance $Z_{tb} = Z_t \times \dfrac{\text{MVA}_b}{\text{MVA}_t}$

$= \dfrac{0.04 \times 10^6}{0.5 \times 10^6} = 0.08$ pu

b.   transformer cable base impedance Zcb, in per unit values, at transformer:

$Z_{cb} = \dfrac{Zc}{Zb} = \dfrac{0.001}{0.17225} = 0.006$ pu

c. total pu value $Z_{tb+cb} = Z_{tb} + Z_{cb} = 0.08 + 0.006$

$$= 0.086 \text{ pu}$$

or stage 2 impedance $Z_2 = Z_{tb+cb} \times Z_b$

$$= 0.086 \times 0.172225 = 0.0148 \text{ ohms.}$$

20.4   The total cumulative impedance up to stage $2 = Z_1 + Z_2$

$$= 0.00156 + 0.0148$$

$$= 0.00164 \text{ ohms,}$$

therefore: total cumulative stage 2 impedance (pu) to the transformer

LV cb $= Z_{cb} + Z_{(tb+cb)}$

$$= 0.009 + 0.086$$

$$= 0.095 \text{ pu}$$

or as cumulative % impedance = 9.5%.

20.5   Actual fault level at the transformer $= \dfrac{10^6}{0.095} = 10.526$ MVA

fault current level $= \dfrac{10.526 \times 10^6}{\sqrt{3} \times 415} = 14.642$ kA.

20.6   The above procedure for stages 3, 4 and 5 may be repeated for all the remaining cable phase impedance ohmic values. The stage cable impedance, divided by the base impedance Z_b, is equal to the stage impedance pu value. The actual fault current level at a stage is found by the sum of the cumulative impedance pu ohmic values previously derived to that stage.

Protection and discrimination

20.7   Figure 19 demonstrates how the simplest protection devices can be arranged to provide adequate discrimination, although the curves shown are only typical of the devices which are available. Designers of protection systems should be able to obtain more truly representative curves for specific devices from the manufacturer. The principle of the HV protection system is applicable to the ring or radial HV main distribution systems shown in Figures 3, 4, 7 and 9. Discrimination between MCBs and fuses is demonstrated. The choice of suitable miniature circuit breakers or moulded case circuit breakers is referred to in paragraph 11.16.

20.8   Table 10 analyses the operating time and the discrimination with back-up devices for three-phase faults at each stage of the typical distribution system. It will be seen that none of the operating times is excessive. Discrimination with back-up devices is adequate except for a fault at point 8, in Figure 19. The 100 A back-up fuse shown was chosen for demonstration purposes only. In practice, a larger fuse (not less than say 160 A) would provide adequate discrimination whilst retaining discrimination with the next stage.

Fault location	Fault level		Operates		Discriminates with	
	kA (415 V base)	MVA	Device	Time(s)	Device	Times(s)
1	0.75	0.54	100A MCCB	0.3	300A fuse	>10
2	1.44	1	100A MCCB	0.1	300A fuse	1
3	1.44	1	300A fuse	1	500A fuse	>10
4	2.6	1.9	300A fuse	0.16	500A fuse	1.6
5	2.6	1.9	500A fuse	1.6	(50A HV fuse)	>10
6	14.6	10.5	500A fuse	<0.1		0.02
7	0.75	0.54	30A MCCB	0.01	100A fuse	0.1
8	1.44	1	30A MCCB	0.01	100A fuse	<.01
9	1.44	1	100A fuse	<0.01	300A fuse	1.0
10	2.6	1.9	100A fuse	<0.01	300A fuse	0.1
11	2.6	1.9	300A fuse	0.16	(50A HV fuse)	>10
12	14.6	10.5	300A fuse	<0.01		0.02
13	14.6	10.5	(50A HV fuse)	0.02	idmt relay	1
14	100*	72		<0.01	idmt relay	0.25
15	154	111		<0.01	idmt relay	0.2
16	154	111	idmt relay	0.2	idmt relay	—

Table 10 Summary of fault levels and operating times of the protective devices shown in Figure 19

21.0 Tariff negotiations and private generation

Regional electricity company agreement

21.1   The REC must make an offer following a request from a private consumer or supplier as required in the provisions of the Energy Act 1983 and Electricity Act 1989:

Electricity (Northern Ireland) Requirements Order 1991

a. for a supply to his premises;

b. to purchase electricity generated by him;

c. to permit him to use the REC system to give a supply to any premises.

It is always essential to carry out close consultation with the REC at the earliest time before embarking on any detailed investigation.

Electricity tariffs

21.2   Each REC has its own series of charges for electricity, and most tariffs which are applicable to HCPs include a maximum demand charge based on twice the maximum number of units supplied during any 30 consecutive minutes within a defined period.

21.3   The most satisfactory schemes have a monthly maximum demand rate which varies from a maximum in winter to a minimum in seven summer months. With this tariff any private generating plant need only operate up to 2000 hours per year, from 1 November until 31 March. These are the times of excess maximum demand in the HCP load.

21.4   For peak lopping or combined heating and power (CHP) schemes, the Regional Electricity Companies will normally make an additional charge for holding available a system standby generating plant capacity. This standby supply is for use only in the event of breakdown and for maintenance of all or part of the private generating plant. The charge is normally expressed in a special tariff, as a system availability charge, negotiated with the consumer in pence per kVA per month of reserved capacity. Availability charges will have an important influence on the overall economics of peak load reduction and CHP savings.

Daily load and annual maximum demand

21.5   When investigating tariffs and/or the possibilities of on-site generation for peak load reduction it is necessary to obtain, in as much detail as possible, the daily, monthly and annual profile of the healthcare premises' electrical and heat demand. For existing HCPs the past electricity and fuel bills will provide the most useful source of information, but for projected HCPs, outline estimates should be used.

21.6   The economic possibility of any peak lopping will not be worthwhile investigating unless the healthcare premises has a peaky load shape which occurs during the winter when the total national load is greater and, hence, when a substantial part of the electricity bill comprises maximum demand charges. The most convenient method to adopt is to calculate the annual load factor. Generally, peak lopping is attractive only for load factors under 30%:

$$\text{Load factor} = \frac{\text{Total power consumed in year/period}}{\text{Total generating capacity installed in year/period.}}$$

21.7   Close attention to methods of improving the annual load factor could be more economically advantageous than peak load reduction.

Cost per unit of generated power

21.8   The cost per unit generated will usually exceed the unit charge of the public supply, and accordingly, an emergency generator should only be used for the periods necessary to achieve the most economic reduction in the maximum demand charge.

21.9   In determining the cost per unit generated it is necessary to take into account the annual plant amortisation cost in addition to the additional cost of fuel, lubrication, labour and maintenance.

21.10   With peak lopping, the consideration must be that the emergency generating plant was provided for emergency purposes only. It is therefore reasonable to assume that the additional cost is related only to such items as involve the additional plant use for peak lopping. This will include such items as bulk fuel storage facilities, synchronising and protection equipment, additional switchgear, contract maximum demand meter, etc that are totally related to parallel running with the Regional electricity company's normal mains supply. If peak lopping entails supplying the designated essential supplies during periods of maximum demand only, these essential supplies being provided entirely from the a.c. emergency generator, the additional cost would relate to larger-capacity fuel oil tanks and increased maintenance and labour charges to maintain the different service of electrical energy.

21.11   For estimating purposes a typical cost per unit generated should be taken as equal to "W" pence, based on fuel oil prices "X" pence per litre and lubricating oil at "Y" pence per litre and an estimated figure of "Z" pence per unit for the foreshortened life of the a.c. emergency generator set, as:

$$W = |X| + |Y| + |Z|$$

Size of generating set

21.12   Regional electricity companies do not discourage small peak lopping schemes in parallel with their system. It should be borne in mind that the additional cost to adapt small plant to peak lopping may not be directly proportional to the rating of the plant size. This is particularly so, considering the additional equipment cost and operating considerations, when parallel running of LV generating plant is being considered. Consequently, it is doubtful if generating sets of less than 250 kW rating for peak lopping would be economic. HTM 2011 – 'Emergency electrical service', considers generating plant in more detail.

21.13   Under the Electricity Act 1989, anyone who generates, transmits or supplies electrical energy will require a licence, unless exempted. Exemption applies to generating sets of less than 10 MW rating and suppliers below 500 kW.

Figures

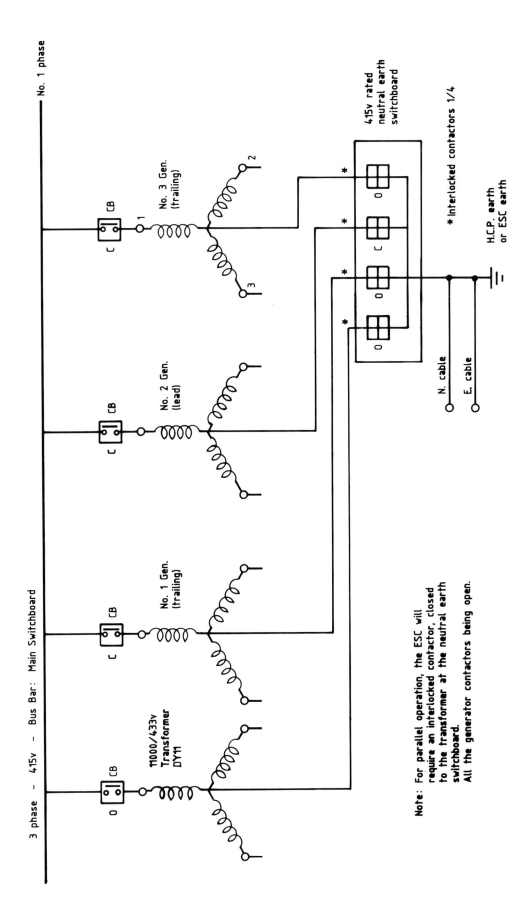

Figure 1 Typical arrangement showing No 2 generator solid earth connection (TN–S) at the neutral earth switchboard for island operation

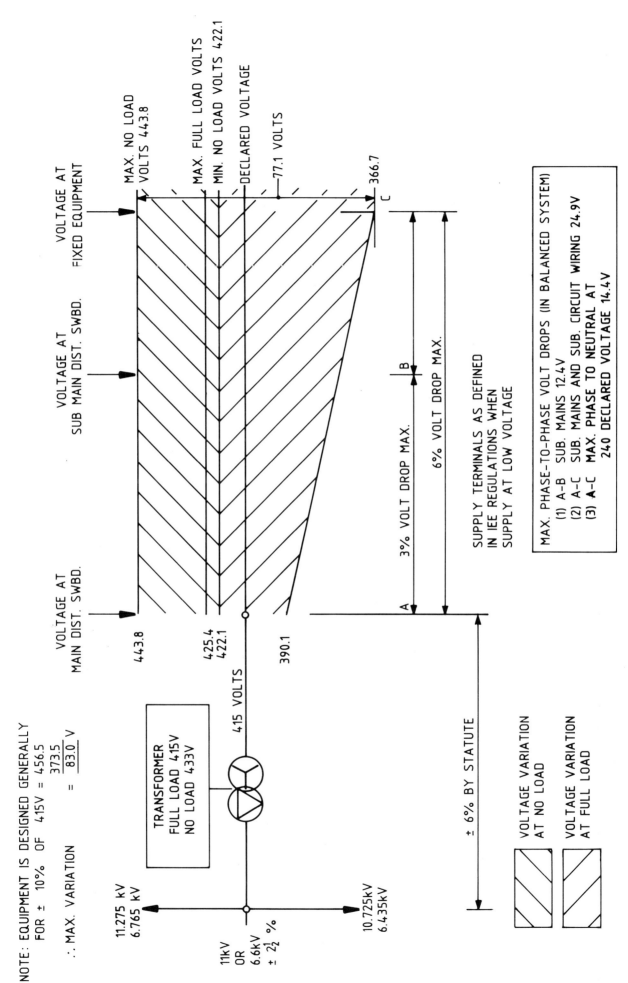

Figure 2 Diagram of voltage variations 415 volt 3 phase 50 cycle

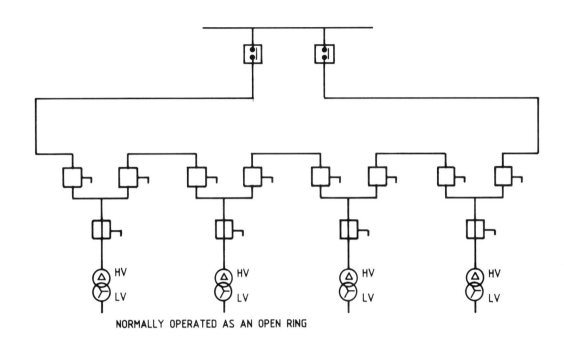

NORMALLY OPERATED AS AN OPEN RING

Figure 3   Typical arrangement of high voltage ring main using ring main units and fused switch protection for transformers

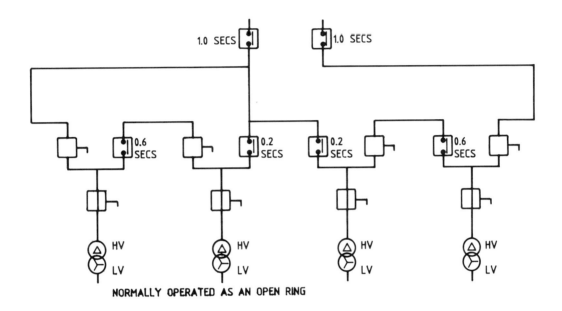

Figure 4 Arrangement of high voltage ring main units with ring isolator, circuit breaker and fused switch protection for transformers with typical protection grading

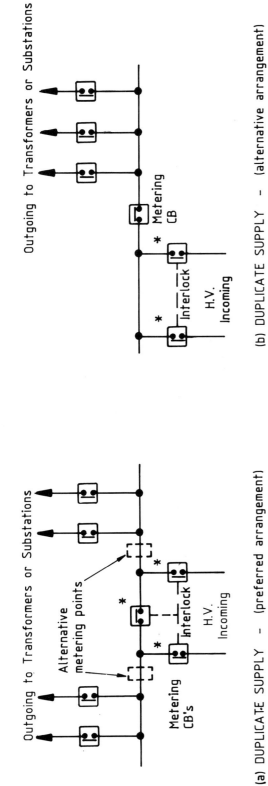

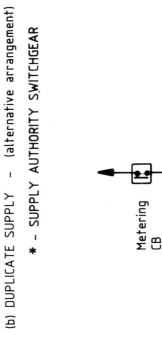

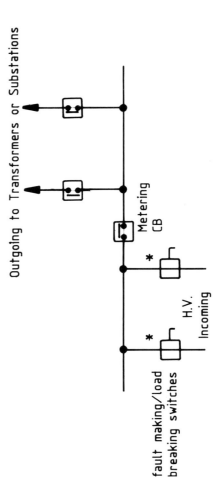

Figure 5 Methods of HV supply and distribution

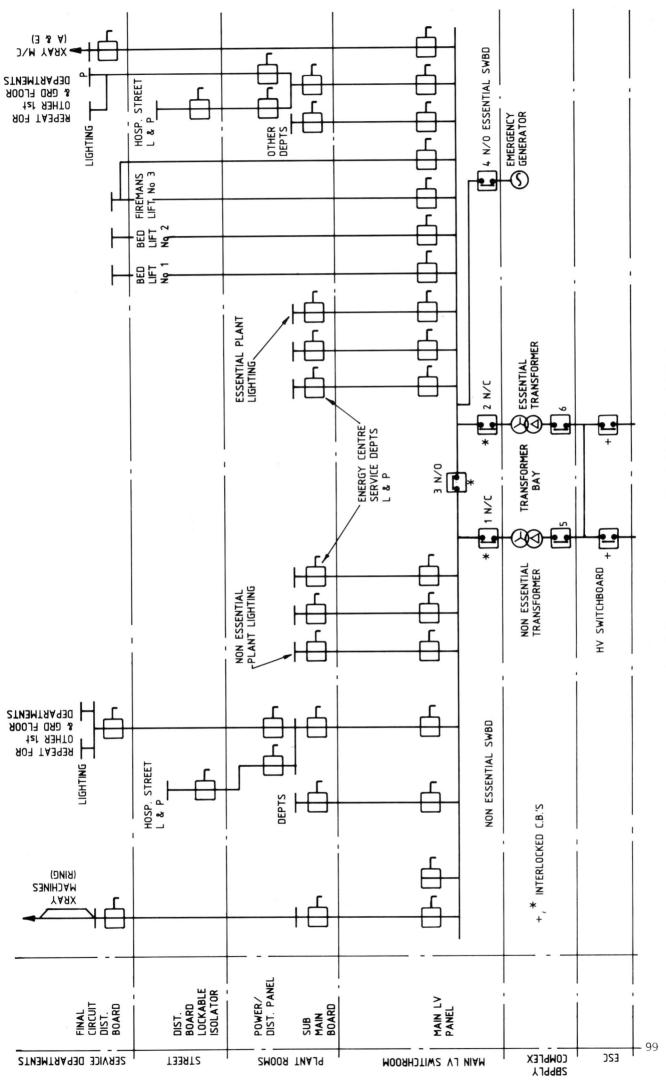

Figure 6 Two-transformer arrangement for electrical supply and distribution

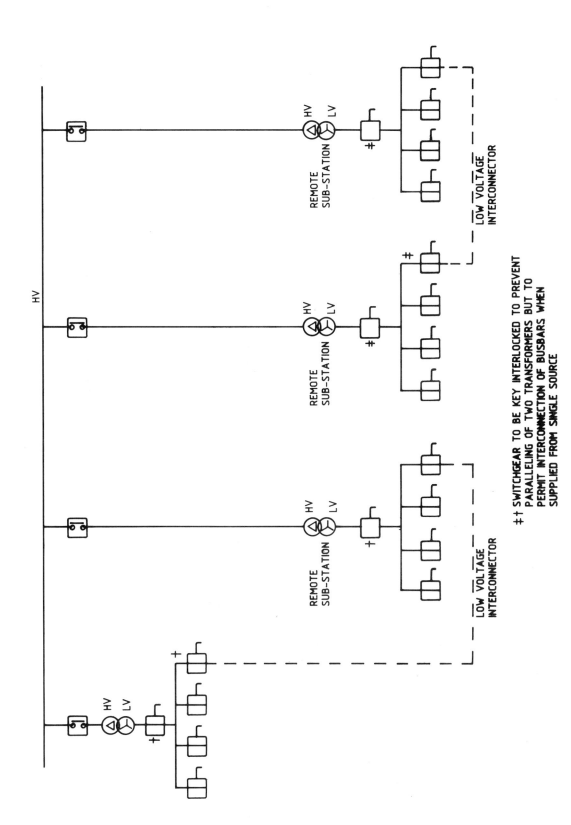

Figure 7   High voltage radial distribution with medium voltage interconnectors

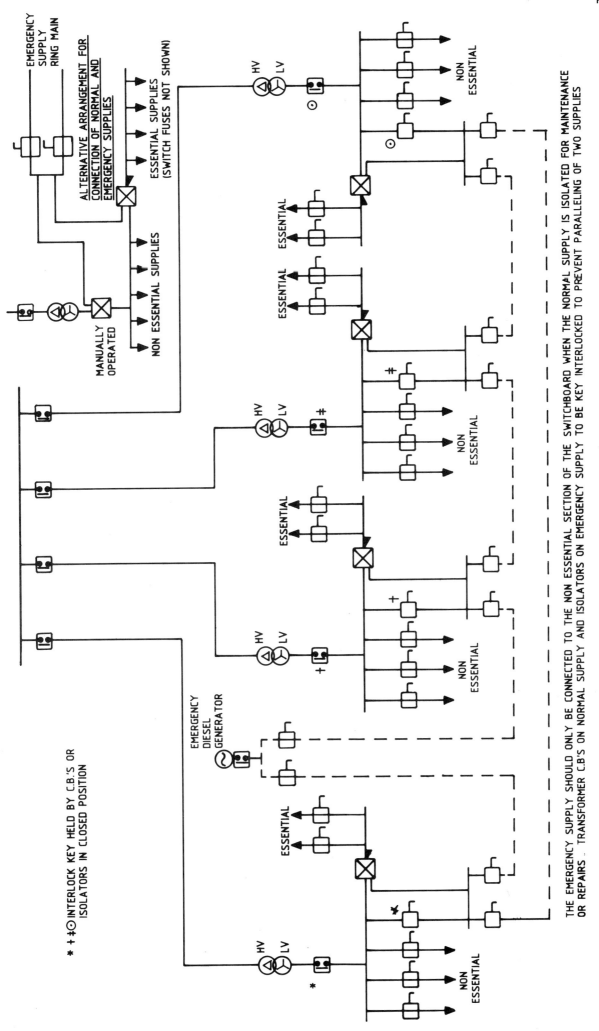

Figure 8 High voltage radial distribution with low voltage emergency ring interconnector

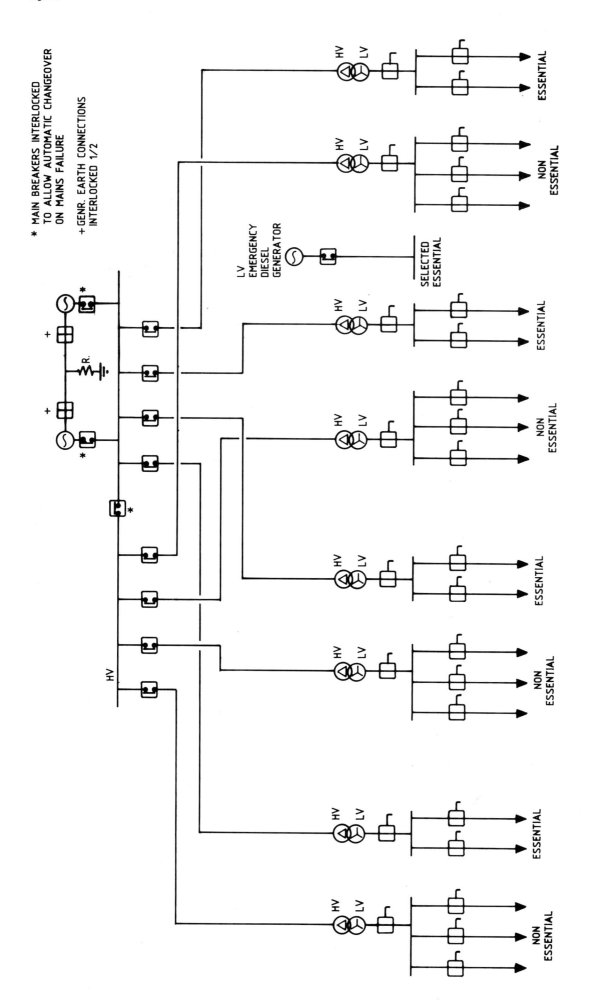

Figure 9   High voltage radial distribution with high voltage generators

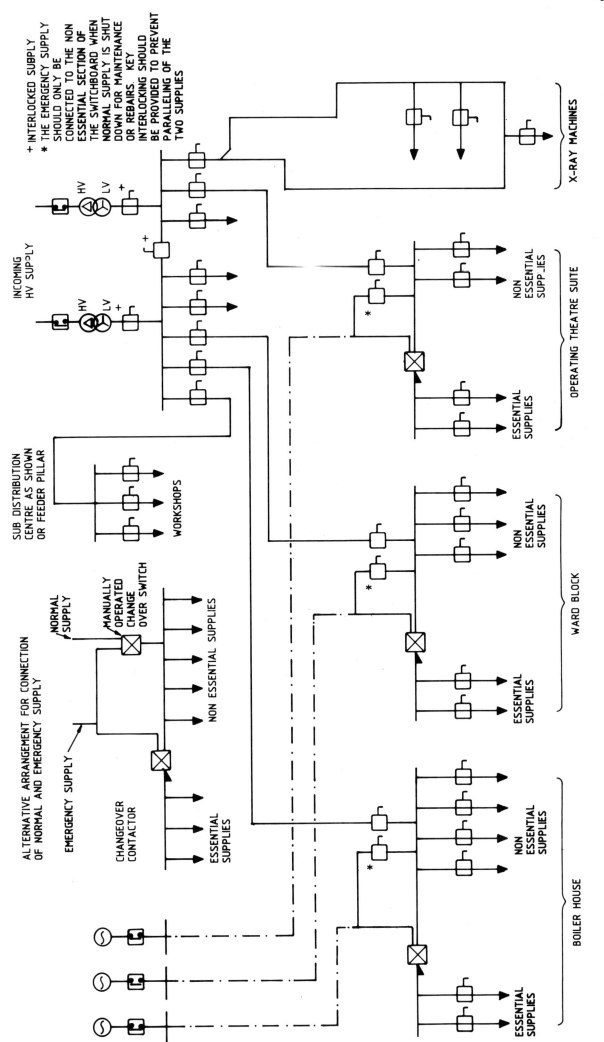

Figure 10 Typical low voltage distribution

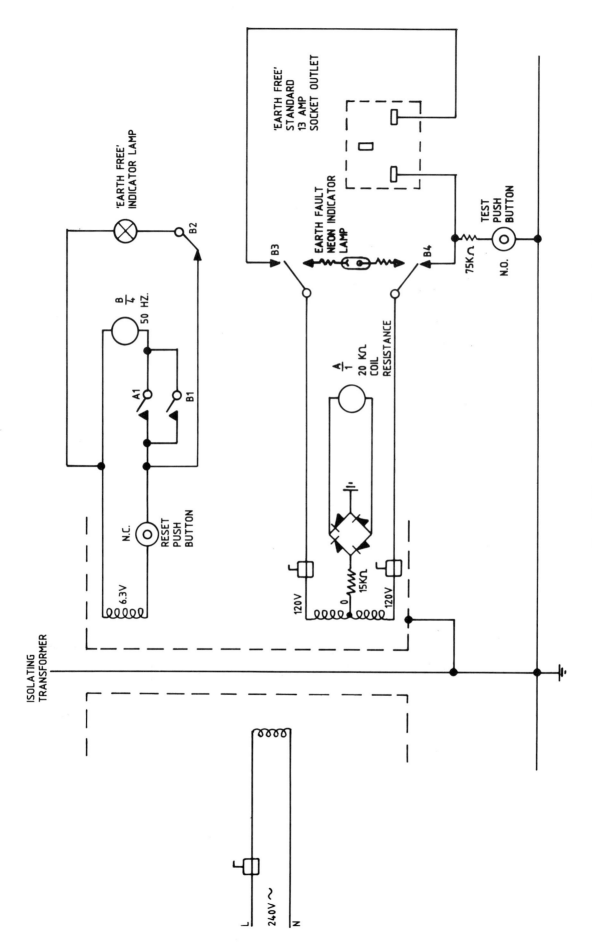

Figure 11 Schematic diagram of an earth free supply unit – post-mortem room

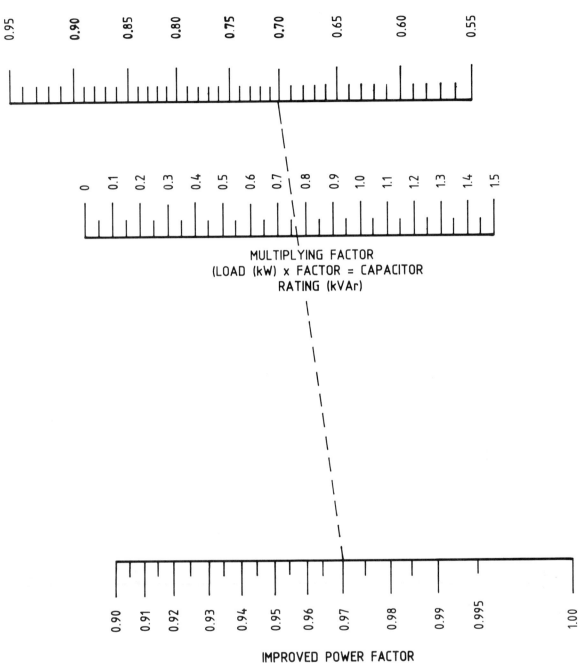

INITIAL POWER FACTOR

MULTIPLYING FACTOR
(LOAD (kW) x FACTOR = CAPACITOR
RATING (kVAr)

IMPROVED POWER FACTOR

Figure 12   Chart for use in determining a power factor improvement capacitor rating

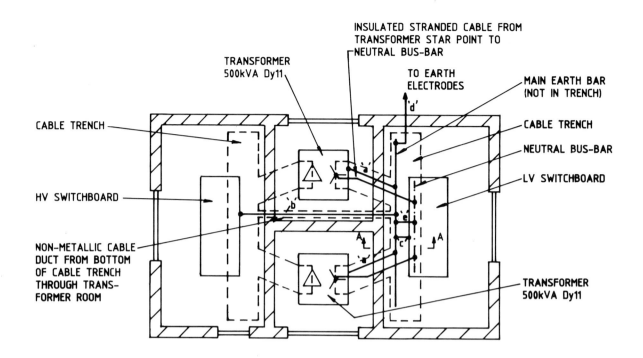

PLAN
FRAME EARTH CONNECTION

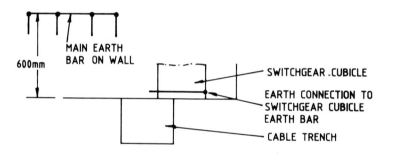

SECTION A–A

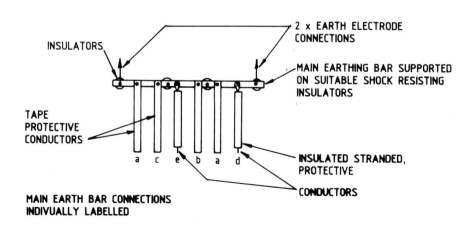

MAIN EARTH BAR CONNECTIONS
INDIVUALLY LABELLED

Figure 13 Sub-station earthing

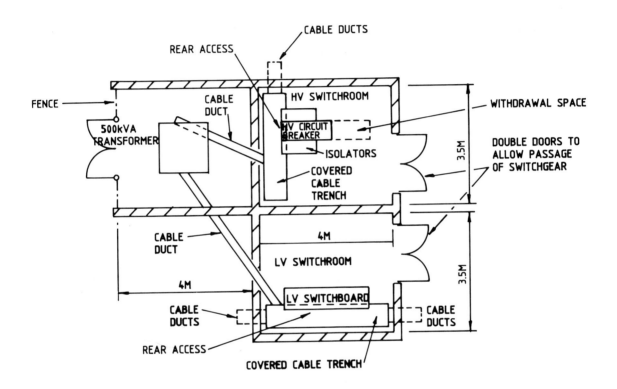

Figure 14 Small sub-station with indoor transformer and high voltage ring main unit switchgear

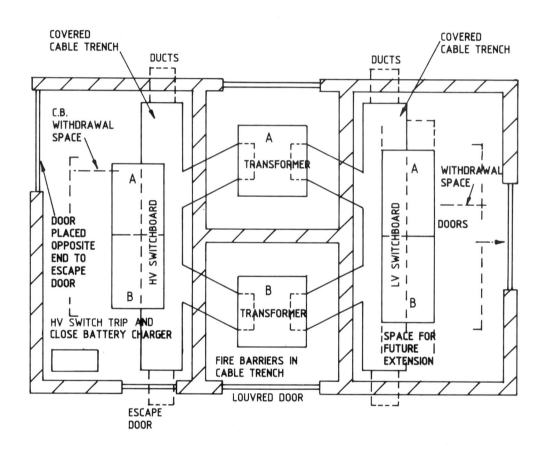

COVERED
CABLE TRENCH

DUCTS

DUCTS

COVERED
CABLE TRENCH

C.B.
WITHDRAWAL
SPACE

A

TRANSFORMER

A

WITHDRAWAL
SPACE

A

DOORS

DOOR
PLACED
OPPOSITE
END TO
ESCAPE
DOOR

HV SWITCHBOARD

LV SWITCHBOARD

HV SWITCH TRIP AND
CLOSE BATTERY CHARGER

B

B

TRANSFORMER

B

SPACE FOR
FUTURE
EXTENSION

FIRE BARRIERS IN
CABLE TRENCH

LOUVRED DOOR

ESCAPE
DOOR

Figure 15   Sub-station with HV ring main switchboard, two transformers and low voltage
switchboard cubicle type

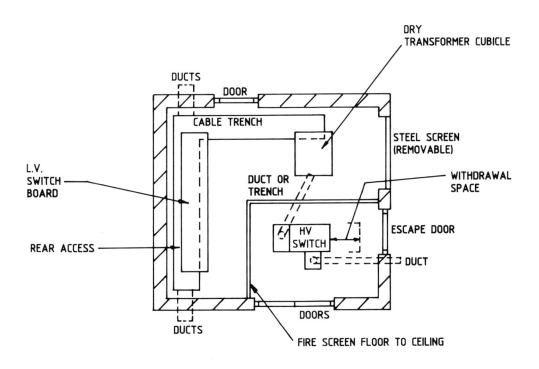

DRY
TRANSFORMER CUBICLE

DUCTS

DOOR

CABLE TRENCH

STEEL SCREEN
(REMOVABLE)

L.V.
SWITCH
BOARD

DUCT OR
TRENCH

WITHDRAWAL
SPACE

HV
SWITCH

ESCAPE DOOR

REAR ACCESS

DUCT

DUCTS

DOORS

FIRE SCREEN FLOOR TO CEILING

PLAN

Figure 16   Sub-station with single HV switch, dry transformer and low voltage switchboard

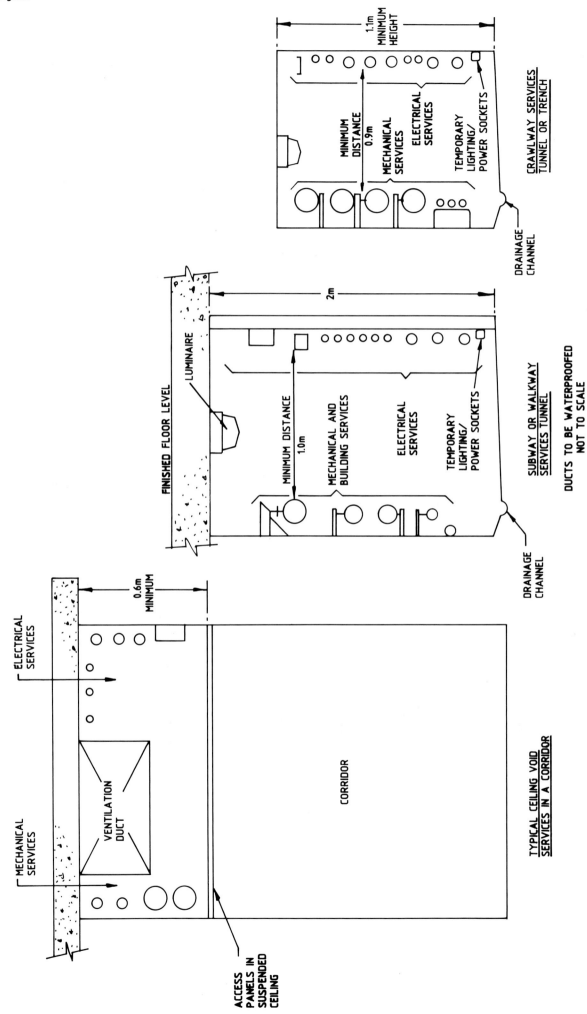

1.1m MINIMUM HEIGHT

MINIMUM DISTANCE 0.9m

MECHANICAL SERVICES

ELECTRICAL SERVICES

TEMPORARY LIGHTING/ POWER SOCKETS

DRAINAGE CHANNEL

CRAWLWAY SERVICES TUNNEL OR TRENCH

FINISHED FLOOR LEVEL

LUMINAIRE

2m

MINIMUM DISTANCE 1.0m

MECHANICAL AND BUILDING SERVICES

ELECTRICAL SERVICES

TEMPORARY LIGHTING/ POWER SOCKETS

DRAINAGE CHANNEL

SUBWAY OR WALKWAY SERVICES TUNNEL

DUCTS TO BE WATERPROOFED NOT TO SCALE

ELECTRICAL SERVICES

0.6m MINIMUM

MECHANICAL SERVICES

VENTILATION DUCT

CORRIDOR

ACCESS PANELS IN SUSPENDED CEILING

TYPICAL CEILING VOID SERVICES IN A CORRIDOR

Figure 17 Typical segregated routes for services

Discrimination and Fault Conditions

1, Figure 19 analyses the 3 phase fault levels which may be expected in a typical H.C.P. distribution circuit from the supply authority intake to the power outlet of the final sub-circuit.

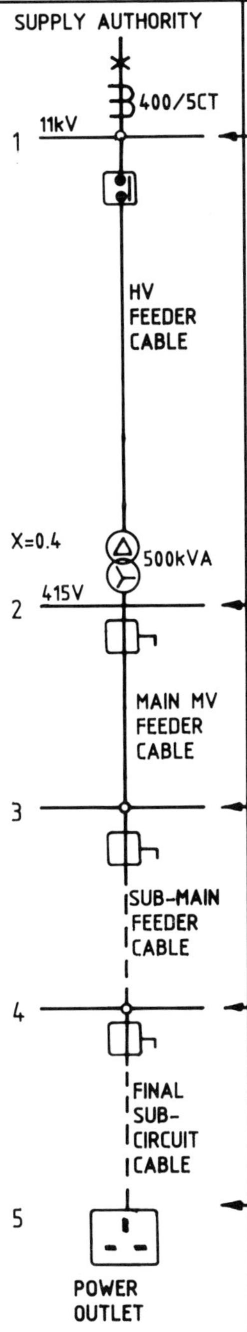

DISTRIBUTION SYSTEM STAGES	STAGE PHASE IMPEDANCE (OHMS)	CUMULATIVE PHASE IMPEDANCE (OHMS)	CUMULATIVE PERCENTAGE IMPEDANCE AT 1MVA BASE	MVA FAULT LEVEL (3 PHASE)	EQUIVALENT kA FAULT LEVEL AT 415 VOLT BASE
SUPPLY AUTHORITY					
1 11kV 400/5CT	0.00156	0.00156	0.9	111.111	154
HV FEEDER CABLE					
X=0.4 500kVA 2 415V	0.0148	0.0164	9.5	10.526	14.642
MAIN MV FEEDER CABLE					
3	0.0751	0.0915	53	1.89	2.63
SUB-MAIN FEEDER CABLE					
4	0.0755	0.167	96.5	1.04	1.44
FINAL SUB-CIRCUIT CABLE					
5	0.153	0.32	185	0.54	0.75
POWER OUTLET					

Figure 18   Typical impedances and fault levels for a healthcare premises distribution network

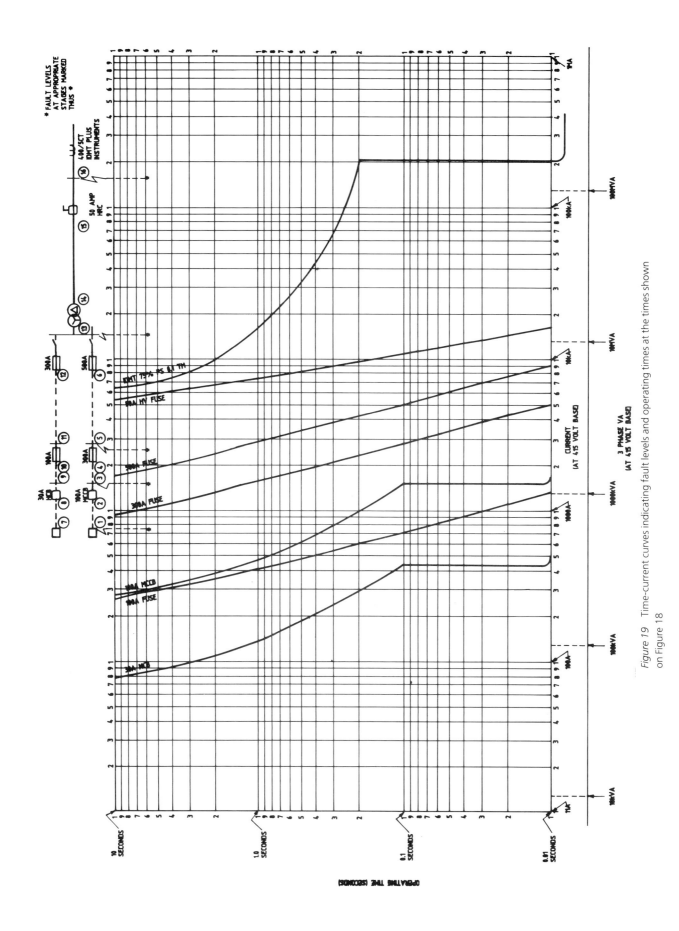

Figure 19 Time-current curves indicating fault levels and operating times at the times shown on Figure 18

Other publications in this series

(Given below are details of all Health Technical Memoranda available from HMSO. HTMs marked (*) are currently being revised, those marked (†) are out of print. Some HTMs in preparation at the time of publication of this HTM are also listed.)

1	Anti-static precautions: rubber, plastics and fabrics*†
2	Anti-static precautions: flooring in anaesthetising areas (and data processing rooms)*, 1977.
3	–
4	–
5	Steam boiler plant instrumentation†
8	–
9	–
10	Sterilizers*†
2011	Emergency electrical services, 1993.
12	–
13	–
2014	Abatement of electrical interference, 1993.
15	Patient/nurse call systems†
16	–
17	Health building engineering installations: commissioning and associated activities, 1978.
18	Facsimile telegraphy: possible applications in DGHs†
19	Facsimile telegraphy: the transmission of pathology reports within a hospital – a case study†
2020	Electrical safety code for low voltage systems, 1993.
2021	Electrical safety code for high voltage systems, 1993.
22	Piped medical gases, medical compressed air and medical vacuum installations*†
22	Supp. Permit to work system: for piped medical gases etc†
23	Access and accommodation for engineering services†
24	–
25	–
26	Commissioning of oil, gas and dual fired boilers: with notes on design, operation and maintenance†
27	Cold water supply storage and mains distribution* [Revised version will deal with water storage and distribution], 1978.
28 to 39	–
2040	The control of legionellae in healthcare premises – a code of practice.
41 to 53	–

Component Data Base (HTMs 54 to 70)

54.1	User manual, 1993.
55	Windows, 1989.
56	Partitions, 1989.
57	Internal glazing, 1989.
58	Internal doorsets, 1989.
59	Ironmongery, 1989.
60	Ceilings, 1989.
61	Flooring, 1989.
62	Demountable storage systems, 1989.
63	Fitted storage systems, 1989.
64	Sanitary assemblies, 1989.
65	Signs†
66	Cubicle curtain track, 1989.
67	Laboratory fitting-out systems, 1993.
68	Ducts and panel assemblies, 1993.
69	Protection, 1993.
70	Fixings, 1993.
71 to 80	–

Firecode

81	Firecode: fire precautions in new hospitals, 1987.
81	Supp 1, 1993
82	Firecode: alarm and detection systems, 1989.
83	Fire safety in health care premises: general fire precautions*†
85	[Revision to Home Office draft guidance in preparation]
86	Firecode: assessing fire risks in existing hospital wards, 1987.
87	Firecode: textiles and furniture, 1993.
88	Fire safety in health care premises: guide to fire precautions in NHS housing in the community for mentally handicapped/ill people, 1986.

New HTMs in preparation

Lifts

Combined heat and power

Telecommunications (telephone exchanges)

Washers for sterile production

Ventilation in healthcare premises

Risk management and quality assurance

Health Technical Memoranda published by HMSO can be purchased from HMSO bookshops in London (post orders to PO Box 276, SW8 5DT), Edinburgh, Belfast, Manchester, Birmingham and Bristol or through good booksellers. HMSO provide a copy service for publications which are out of print; and a standing order service.

Enquiries about Health Technical Memoranda (but not orders) should be addressed to: NHS Estates, Department of Health, Publications and Marketing Unit, 1 Trevelyan Square, Boar Lane, Leeds LS1 6AE.

About NHS Estates

NHS Estates is an Executive Agency of the Department of Health and is involved with all aspects of health estate management, development and maintenance. The Agency has a dynamic fund of knowledge which it has acquired during 30 years of working in the field. Using this knowledge NHS Estates has developed products which are unique in range and depth. These are described below.

NHS Estates also makes its experience available to the field through its consultancy services.

Enquiries should be addressed to: NHS Estates, Department of Health, 1 Trevelyan Square, Boar Lane, Leeds LS1 6AE. Tel: 0532 547000.

Some other NHS Estates products

Activity DataBase – a computerised system for defining the activities which have to be accommodated in spaces within health buildings. *NHS Estates*

Design Guides – complementary to Health Building Notes, Design Guides provide advice for planners and designers about subjects not appropriate to the Health Building Notes series. *HMSO*

Estatecode – user manual for managing a health estate. Includes a recommended methodology for property appraisal and provides a basis for integration of the estate into corporate business planning. *HMSO*

Capricode – a framework for the efficient management of capital projects from inception to completion. *HMSO*

Concode – outlines proven methods of selecting contracts and commissioning consultants. Both parts reflect official policy on contract procedures. *HMSO*

Works Information Management System – a computerised information system for estate management tasks, enabling tangible assets to be put into the context of servicing requirements. *NHS Estates*

Option Appraisal Guide – advice during the early stages of evaluating a proposed capital building scheme. Supplementary guidance to Capricode. *HMSO*

Health Building Notes – advice for project teams procuring new buildings and adapting or extending existing buildings. *HMSO*

Health Facilities Notes – debate current and topical issues of concern across all areas of healthcare provision. *HMSO*

Health Guidance Notes – an occasional series of publications which respond to changes in Department of Health policy or reflect changing NHS operational management. Each deals with a specific topic and is complementary to a related Health Technical Memorandum. *HMSO*

Encode – shows how to plan and implement a policy of energy efficiency in a building. *HMSO*

Firecode – for policy, technical guidance and specialist aspects of fire precautions. *HMSO*

Nucleus – standardised briefing and planning system combining appropriate standards of clinical care and service with maximum economy in capital and running costs. *NHS Estates*

Concise – software support for managing the capital programme. Compatible with Capricode. *NHS Estates*

Items noted "HMSO" can be purchased from HMSO bookshops in London (post orders to PO Box 276, SW8 5DT), Edinburgh, Belfast, Manchester, Birmingham and Bristol or through good booksellers. Details of their standing order service are given at the front of this publication.

Enquiries about NHS Estates products should be addressed to: NHS Estates, Marketing and Publications Unit, Department of Health, 1 Trevelyan Square, Boar Lane, Leeds LS1 6AE.

NHS Estates consultancy service

Designed to meet a range of needs from advice on the oversight of estates management functions to a much fuller collaboration for particularly innovative or exemplary projects.

Enquiries should be addressed to: NHS Estates, Consultancy Service (address as above).

Printed in the United Kingdom for HMSO.
Dd.297556 C 15 11/93